Fighting Lupus Battles:
Hope For A Cure

True Stories From Lupus Warriors

Kayrene Mimms

Hilton Publishing · Chicago, Illinois

Hilton Publishing Company
Chicago, IL

Direct all correspondence to:
Hilton Publishing Company
1630 45th St. Suite B101
Munster, IN 46321
(219) 922–4868
www.hiltonpub.com

ISBN 978-0-9904283-2-9

Notice: The information in this book is true and complete to the best knowledge of the author and publisher. This book is intended only as an informational reference and should not replace, countermand, or conflict with the advice given to readers by their physicians. The author and publisher disclaim all liability in connection with the specific personal use of any and all information provided in this book. You should consult with a professional where appropriate. Neither the publisher nor author shall be liable for any loss of profit or any other damages, including but not limited to special, incidental, consequential, or other damages.

Printed in the United States of America.

Publisher & Director of Production/Editorial: Megan Lippert
Senior Book Design/Editorial: Angela Vennemann

Photographs & images provided by Author and Contributing Chapter Authors

Cover photo is copyright © 2011 by Thomas Park and made available under a Creative Commons Attribution 2.0 license. https://creativecommons.org/licenses/by/2.0/. The cover photo was flipped horizontally from the original version, and text was added.

Library of Congress Cataloging-in-Publication Data

Mimms, Kayrene, compiler.
    Fighting lupus battles : hope for a cure : true stories from lupus warriors / [compiled by] Kayrene Mimms.
        p.   ; cm.
    Includes bibliographical references.
    ISBN 978-0-9904283-2-9
    I. Title.
    [DNLM: 1. Lupus Erythematosus, Systemic—Personal Narratives. 2. Survivors—Personal Narratives. WD 380]
    RC924.5.L85
    616.7′72—dc23
                        2015018245

Dedication

For my nieces, Noel and Belinda, along with all those patients who, because they did not receive an accurate and timely lupus diagnosis, suffered devastating health issues that were too far advanced to survive.

Contents

Acknowledgements

I am very grateful to all who gave of their time and helped in bringing this project to completion. Fellow lupus patients and their family members have shared the most intimate details about their journey with lupus. Lupus patients, relatives, and medical professionals who wrote stories for this book are: Tari Ambler; Robinzina Bryant, retired FBI special agent; Sherron N. Buford; Lois Burleson; Jocelyn O. Carreón; Ashley Chappell-Rice; Collette Clark; Brandi L. Collins; Erica M. Collins, PhD; H.L. Collins; Ivy M. Douglas; Helena Fields; Jameela Lindsey; Richard Mebane; Cecil Mimms, Jr.; Celia Mimms, DDS; Kayrene Mimms; Carla Y. Moore, MS, CCC-SLP; Chenise G. Rias; Kelley Rose; Patricia L. Sanders; Sarah Spadoni, CVT; Kanefus R. Walker; and Michael Zielinski, MD, FACP.

I express special thanks to attorneys David C. Hilliard and Andrew R.W. Hughes of Pattishall, McAuliffe, Newbury, Hilliard & Geraldson LLP for providing countless hours of pro bono legal advice. I am ever so grateful to Rosalind Ramsey-Goldman, MD, DrPH for providing a medical perspective and teaching points for our readers. I would also like to express my sincere appreciation to my supporters who provided encouragement, inspiration, editing, review, and recommendations. They include: Charles Brummell, President/CEO of the Lupus Society of Illinois; Monica Fountain of The Well magazine; Dr. Anthony Gantt; Virginia A. Mitamura; Patricia A. Murphy, MSN, CNP, CNM; Lewis Nixon; Janice M. Stewart; Dr. Caroloretta Tucker; Bernard C. Turner; and Sarah Wallace-Crawley, RN, PNP, Ed.D. I sincerely thank Dr. Hilton M. Hudson, II, President/CEO of Hilton Publishing Company (HPC), for accepting my proposal. Also thanks to Megan Lippert and Angela Vennemann of HPC who patiently walked me through the publishing process.

Author's Disclaimer

The purpose of this book, *Fighting Lupus Battles: Hope For a Cure*, is to increase lupus awareness. I am not a medical professional and do not claim to be an expert in lupus in any way. Rather, I am an individual who has been diagnosed with lupus, who wants to share my story and the stories of other lupus patients with the world. The participants have guaranteed that their stories represent factual accounts of their experiences. We provide this information to help shed light on the complexity of this disease, not to offer any professional advice or services.

The scientific information about lupus definition, types, symptoms, diagnosis, and research is taken from publications provided by the Lupus Foundation of America, Inc. (LFA), the Lupus Society of Illinois (LSI), the National Institute of Arthritis and Musculoskeletal and Skin Diseases (NIAMS), and the National Institutes of Health (NIH). The author and other participants shall not be held liable or responsible to any person or entity for loss or damage caused or alleged to be caused directly or indirectly by the information contained in this book. If anyone has any of the symptoms that are discussed, we recommend that you seek professional medical advice as soon as possible.

Foreword

Fighting Lupus Battles: Hope For a Cure by Kayrene Mimms is written clearly to inform patients, families, friends, and allied health personnel about a very provocative disease. The author has succeeded in providing riveting stories woven into an intriguing, informative, in-depth guide through the individual voices of lupus patients in an understanding and empathetic manner. Sometimes is it difficult to find an interesting book on a little known disease that will have you spellbound to the point you cannot stop reading. After having read the book a second time, I found myself perusing the stories, and was amazed at how each of the characters' lives were strangely interwoven with the others, and how they evolved and blended into the flow of the main topic of lupus. This must-read and reassuring book also provides easy practical resources, tips, and a quiz to round out information for the reader's understanding.

Sarah Wallace-Crawley, RN, PNP, EdD

School Nurse/Pediatric Nurse Practitioner, Chicago Public Schools/Chicago Health Department

✶✶✶✶✶✶

Fighting Lupus Battles: Hope For a Cure is a collection of stories that immediately captures your attention. The stories bring lupus to life and give the reader a small peek into the challenges and suffering incurred by individuals with lupus on a daily basis.

Many people with lupus suffer for years before receiving a correct diagnosis. During that time, lupus, which is unpredictable, can show itself in many ways, from impacting the joints and skin to impacting the vital organs.

Be prepared, as you read these stories, to feel the personal side of lupus.

Charles Brummell

President/CEO, Lupus Society of Illinois

****

This is a very good read! I could not put it down. It's knowledge. It's about personal journeys. It's an invitation to WAR on lupus.

Several years ago I met lupus on my way to another normal day in my life. My very dear friend experienced a lupus crisis which resulted in sixty-five days in Chicago's Northwestern Hospital's Intensive Care Unit followed by months of rehab. I had always seen her as a healthy, active woman of substance. Lupus challenged everything I knew about her but also provided an atmosphere conducive to learning. I not only learned about the disease, but how truly resilient my friend and others are who face lupus challenges on a daily basis.

This book provides the reader an opportunity to gain knowledge about lupus; the disease, the patients, treatment options and impact to family members and friends. Woven throughout the pages are explanations of symptoms, personal heartfelt stories of coping, and awareness that lupus, to date, is an undefeated enemy. But there is also hope.

Let's declare war on lupus by continuing to educate ourselves while providing various forms of support to patients and their families—those on the front lines—and continuing to raise funds. Through research, a cure can be found.

Janice M. Stewart

****

It has been a privilege to be part of the rheumatology team caring for Ms. Kay Mimms since 2008. I have witnessed firsthand the support and devotion of her husband Cecil, who is with her at almost every appointment. Kay, her husband, and I work as a team to manage her illness. As she mentions in her book, Kay brings a list of notes and questions to every visit for us to review together. At the end of every list she writes that she is living well with lupus.

I feel strongly that one of the reasons she lives well with lupus is due to the support she receives from her family, friends, and the support group. She has provided support to a number of people who have been newly diagnosed with lupus and is always willing to have a fellow patient call her. I have received many positive comments from patients who have spoken to Kay and/or gone to the support group.

As a care provider, it was a humbling experience to read her story as well as those of other lupus patients. Everyone—patients, family and caregivers—who are touched by lupus continue to hope that we will one day find a cure for this disease.

Patricia A. Murphy, MSN, CNP, CNM

****

It is an honor and a privilege that Mrs. Mimms asked me to read her book. When I offered to write a commentary for her book, she and the publisher embraced the idea. My goals for this commentary are several-fold. I want to maintain the lupus patients' voices while clarifying medical concepts. I hope to clarify some of the medical issues encountered by patients with lupus, and I want to provide teaching points that will help in understanding the patients' stories. I will also illustrate how patients and families hear information from healthcare providers but may not get the correct facts, even if the health care provider's intention is to educate and support. (An example of this type of problem is how a skin biopsy was interpreted as a skin graft). This illustrates another reason why lupus patients need to educate themselves about their disease.

These are the themes highlighted in the commentary for each of the stories that lupus survivors and their families have shared in this book:

- Delays and difficulties in making the diagnosis of lupus
- Learning how to minimize flares
- Learning as much as you can about lupus from mild to severe problems
- Research is needed to find better treatment, to prevent disease damage, and ultimately prevent the disease itself
- Learning how to cope
- Learning how to maintain a healthy life style while you have a chronic illness

- Learning how to be an advocate
- Support systems
- Damage from disease and/or treatment
- A lupus patient can look normal but feel bad.
- Pregnancy presents special challenges.
- Other medical problems can occur when you have lupus.
- Impact of disease on work life, friends and family life
- Applying for disability

I hope these additional comments will broaden your understanding of this disease, help you and your healthcare provider manage this disease together, help you to be a better advocate for yourself and for those who suffer from lupus, and encourage you to support research as we learn more about this disease and strive for a cure.

Rosalind Ramsey-Goldman, MD, DrPH
Solovy Arthritis Research Society
Research Professor of Medicine/Rheumatology

Dr. Ramsey-Goldman wrote comments and teaching points for each patient's story. Her commentary can be found at the end of Part 4, on page 160.

Introduction

Lupus is an autoimmune disease. Instead of the immune system protecting the body, it becomes overactive and attacks healthy tissues and organs in the body. According to the National Institutes of Health (NIH), an overactive immune system causes damage to various body tissues and organs. Therefore, lupus can affect many parts of the body, including the blood vessels, brain, heart, joints, kidneys, lungs, and skin.

It seems that most people know very little about lupus. You say lupus, and you get mixed reactions. Some people give you a blank stare and ask, "What is it?" Some immediately start talking about how they know or knew someone with lupus. I always listen carefully for the verb—know or knew—and then I usually repeat the tense they used. That way I can determine if the person they are referring to is still alive. Some might reveal a few things they've heard about the causes and symptoms. Many times I discover that their perception is not reflective of the research. Some might reveal how they believed the one who had been diagnosed with lupus was lazy. They might admit that they just didn't understand and didn't know what to do to help the person.

This book, *Fighting Lupus Battles: Hope For a Cure*, consists of true stories that were written by lupus patients and their relatives. The stories describe the struggles, losses, and victories experienced by us and were written to inspire, encourage, and increase awareness. I want readers to hear from those who have dealt with this complex disease. I hope that as you read these stories, you will become more aware of what it's *really* like dealing with lupus. I also hope that the stories will motivate you to become more involved in helping to educate the public and promote more recognition, respect, notoriety, and importance for the lupus cause. This, in turn, will help us move toward creating more reliable and less damaging treatment plans. The ultimate objective is to move toward discovering a cure for this cruel and peculiar disease called lupus.

The Lupus Society of Illinois (LSI) estimates that there are 5 million people in the world, 1.5 million in the United States, and 65,000 in Illinois who struggle with some form of lupus. Come with me as we learn more about the journeys of a few lupus patients who live in The Prairie State of Illinois.

Part 1

What is Lupus?

Like so many others, I am a lupus patient trying to gain knowledge about my condition. I'm not a medical professional, but I feel it's important and worthwhile to share that information and my personal lupus experience with others suffering from this disease. That's why in 2013–2014, I pulled together all the information I could find on lupus. Information was gathered from various written materials and websites of the following organizations: the American College of Rheumatology (ACR), the Centers for Disease Control and Prevention (CDC), Lupus Foundation of America, Inc. (LFA), Lupus Society of Illinois (LSI), National Institute of Arthritis and Musculoskeletal and Skin Diseases (NIAMS), and National Institutes of Health (NIH).

What follows in Part 1 of this book is a summary of the material I researched along with two stories that reveal some of my personal experiences with lupus.

The Elusive Enemy

by Kay Mimms

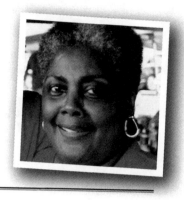

Aheavy coat was a good idea on this windy, cloudy, and cold day in November as we were being driven to the airport. I could dump the coat later because we would soon experience the sunny, hot climate of the Caribbean. The cruise ship would be ready to take us on a wonderful fourteen-day adventure to various islands, through the Panama Canal, and along the coasts of Mexico and California.

I was really looking forward to this trip. Hot weather always made my bones, joints, and muscles feel much better, and this time I had been suffering a lot. I was tired all the time, and the pain in my joints and muscles was almost unbearable. One day Celia, our younger daughter, watched me as I tackled the stairs. She said, "Mom, you look like an old woman." My answer was, "I *feel* like an old woman." Even with the pain and fatigue, I still dragged myself to the health club at least three days a week. I'd do Generation Aqua, Gentle Yoga, or Silver Cycling, thinking that these would help me get better. I was so tired that I would barely make it home, and as soon as I got home, I would collapse on the sofa and sleep for hours. Sometimes I would begin fixing dinner and would have to turn the oven or stove off and take a nap. I never wanted to eat because food tasted either like nothing or like what I thought metal would taste like. I was losing weight fast. I liked the weight loss thing, but I knew it wasn't a healthy form of weight loss.

One night on the cruise, my family and I were having dinner. After dinner, I stood to go to our cabin and discovered that I could barely move my legs. I held on to Cecil, my husband, as we slowly made our way to our cabin. The cabin felt extremely cold to me, and my joints and muscles hurt as if I had been hit by a truck. I dressed in layers of nightwear and a heavy robe, took some aspirin, hiked the thermostat up to 80 degrees (I felt sorry for poor Cecil, who loves a cold room), put my feet under pillows, and got under all the blankets that were in our cabin.

I don't think I had ever felt so cold or experienced such throbbing pain as I did all through that night. I finally fell asleep in the wee hours of the morning and felt better when I woke up for the day. During the remainder of the cruise, I tried to stay as warm as possible. Little did I know at the time that being exposed to lots of sun and high heat might not have been the best thing for me.

After the cruise, we were determined to find out what was wrong with me, so my primary care physician aggressively sought answers. She listened to all my complaints and had me complete all sorts of tests. They included a stress test, colonoscopy, thyroid scan, bone density scan, upper gastrointestinal series, a very painful bone marrow biopsy, various blood tests, and MRIs of my shoulders, arms, and knees. She was very thorough.

I began having more problems with my skin. My cheeks started to lighten; the shape of the discoloration looked like a butterfly. The whites of one of my eyes had reddish streaks. I had experienced both of these conditions throughout the years, but not necessarily at the same time. On recommendations from my dermatologist and ophthalmologist, my primary doctor also evaluated me for lupus. Each one of my doctors suspected I had lupus, yet the results of their evaluations failed to show enough markers for a definitive lupus diagnosis. Therefore, my primary doctor kept searching and trying to solve the mystery of my complaints and deteriorating health condition.

On Christmas day, we made our usual plans of hosting the family dinner. I was still having aches and pains and had learned to take more naps to combat the fatigue. We completed some preparations in the morning so that I could nap for a couple of hours before other family members arrived for our 4:00 p.m. family dinner. So around 1:00 p.m., I lay down for my nap. When I woke up, I felt refreshed and energetic enough to finish the last-minute dinner preparations. I went downstairs and announced, "Let's finish getting ready for the family dinner." Cecil looked at me in a strange way and said, "We've already eaten." All thirty or so family members had eaten, cleaned up, and started to enjoy our usual after-dinner activities. I was really outdone. That's when we all realized that something was terribly wrong because I had napped for over four hours.

Our cousin, Dr. Alfred Cook, was one of my family members who expressed special concern for my condition. He referred me to one of his colleagues, Dr. Michael Zielinski, who apparently loved to research medical puzzles. Dr. Zielinski reviewed my medical history and had me undergo many laboratory tests. After researching my medical history and lab results, he concluded that I have systemic lupus erythematosus (SLE), what is generally referred to as lupus. However, before I was able to secure an appointment with a lupus specialist, my condition suddenly and rapidly worsened. I ended up being sedated and intubated in intensive care for more than two months. That was 2006, and I was 59 years old.

What is lupus?

The National Institutes of Health (NIH) describes lupus as a complex, lifelong, mysterious, and potentially devastating autoimmune disease.[1] Lupus is identified as an autoimmune disease because the body attacks itself. "A healthy immune system produces proteins . . . that help fight and destroy viruses, bacteria, and other foreign substances that invade the body."[2]

If one has lupus, the immune system becomes overactive and also attacks healthy tissues. Cells that are supposed to protect the body from disease end up assaulting the healthy organs and tissues of the body.

According to the NIH, any part of the body can be affected by lupus, including the kidneys, lungs, central nervous system, blood vessels, blood, and heart.[3] "Lupus is unpredictable because it is a disease of flares (symptoms worsen and you feel ill) and remissions (symptoms improve and you feel better)."[4] Health effects of lupus might include, but are not limited to, heart attacks, strokes, seizures, kidney failure, and miscarriages.[5]

What causes lupus?

Though the exact causes of lupus are unknown, many scientists believe that lupus develops as a response to a combination of internal and external factors including hormones, genetics, and the environment.[6] Scientists also report evidence that specific triggers like sunlight, stress, and certain medicines may cause some people to experience lupus flares.[7] According to the American College of Rheumatology, "Most often, lupus starts in people in their 20s and 30s. It occurs ten times more often in women than in men."[8]

"Anyone can get lupus, but it most often affects women. Lupus is also more common in women of African American, Hispanic, Asian, and Native American descent than in Caucasian women."[9]

Is there more than one type of lupus?

The NIH describes several forms of lupus that affect the body in various ways for various reasons at various stages of life.[10]

- **Systemic lupus erythematosus (SLE)** is what most people are referring to when they say lupus. The symptoms may be mild or serious, and any tissue or organ may be affected.
- With **discoid lupus erythematosus (DLE)**, the skin has a red, raised rash that may become thick, scaly, and scarred.
- **Subacute cutaneous lupus erythematosus** presents as skin lesions on parts of the body that are exposed to the sun. Scarring is usually not part of the disease process.
- **Drug-induced lupus erythematosus (DILE)** "is a form of lupus caused by medications ... Symptoms are similar to SLE ... and they typically go away completely when the drug is stopped."
- **Neonatal lupus (NL)** "is a rare disease that can occur in newborn babies."

What are the most common symptoms?

"Each person with lupus has slightly different symptoms that can range from mild to severe and may come and go over time."[11] Some possible symptoms for lupus patients include: abnormal blood clotting; anemia; butterfly-shaped rash across cheeks and nose; extreme fatigue and weakness; fingers turning white and/or blue when cold; frequent fevers with no cause; headaches; low white blood count; pain in chest on deep breathing; sun- or light-sensitivity; swelling in the ankles, feet, glands, hands, legs, and around the eyes; swollen, achy joints and muscles; skin rashes, most often on the face; sores in the mouth and nose; and unexplained hair loss. Patients usually don't display all these symptoms. LSI suggests that individuals who have any of these symptoms should talk to their doctor about lupus. Early diagnosis and proper medical care are very important in managing lupus.

Is lupus easy to diagnose?

Lupus can take months, sometimes years, to be diagnosed. Some common tools that are used to diagnose lupus include a patient's medical history, a complete physical examination, laboratory tests, x-rays, and other imaging tests.[12] "Because symptoms vary from person to person, can come and go over time, and mimic other illnesses, lupus can be difficult to diagnose—and there is no definitive test for lupus."[13]

The Wake

by Kay Mimms

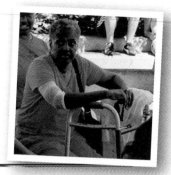

Life has presented me with many unusual situations, but I never thought I would come so close to dying before the age of sixty. I keep thinking about the dreams, hallucinations, and half realities I had when I was intubated and sedated in the intensive care unit for sixty-five days. There were the two wakes, the candle-lighting and washing ceremony, visiting my aunt and obese/paralyzed cousin in Philly, my mother-in-law's visit, and others. Tonight all the images flood my brain and prevent my falling into a restful state of mind. My thoughts settle on the dream of my death or killing session.

Cecil and our older daughter, Carla, are planning a wake for me. They order the food, which is very expensive since a lot of people are expected. After all, there are members of our church groups, retirement groups, health clubs, line dance classes, card playing groups, LSI committees, and all our family members.

Carla is concerned about the potential crowd. She says to Cecil, "Pops, Mom would not forgive us if we ran out of food; you know how she is about making sure there's enough for everyone."

Cecil responds, "But I'm not trying to provide a full-course meal. We should just give them cookies and punch anyway." There is a deep breath from Cecil. Then he says, "All right, just go ahead and order what you want."

My death is scheduled for 6:00 p.m. on Tuesday, so they plan the wake for 7:00 p.m. the same day. My thought is, *"Man, they're not wasting any time!"*

Promptly, at 5:30 p.m., the death technician (DT) comes to my room and takes me to the killing room in the basement of the hospital. He prepares me, then he arranges the equipment. At 5:45 p.m., he applies the killing shock. Surprisingly, it doesn't work. He checks out the equipment and tries again. It still doesn't work. Though he knows I'm not able to respond in any way, I hear him say to me, "Time's up, Kay. You're not cooperating. You won't die. So that's it. Either they cancel the planned death and you live, or they have to plan another killing session."

Cecil is frustrated upon hearing the news that the killing shock didn't work. It's not that he wants me to die; he is distraught that I have to experience death this way. People are arriving for the wake, eating all the food, drinking all the pop and punch, but there is no corpse for the wake. I'm still alive.

Of course, everyone wants me to live; at least, I think so. But the doctors say I can't live in my state, and I need to be put to death. So they have to reschedule the death and the wake. Cecil is really upset now. Not only do I have to go through the killing session again, but they also have to plan and pay for another wake and entertain all those people. (Anyone who knows Cecil will recognize one of his deeply entrenched attributes—frugality.) Cecil is thinking, "Why do we have to do this twice? Why does Kay have to be put to death anyway? Death should be a calm and peaceful transition, not the result of a surging bolt of electricity."

They plan another event for a few days later. On the day of the wake, the DT is pushing my bed down the hallway. I see the ceiling lights, the exit signs, the tops of doors, creases between the ceilings and walls, the emergency switches, and finally the room with the large circular florescent lamp that can be tilted if needed. The table can also be tilted. In fact, it seems to be floating and tilting to reach a certain position. The DT finally seems to be satisfied with the position of the table and pushes a button to stop the motion. He checks his protective gear and his equipment one last time. He attaches the equipment to me and activates the controls. I hear the noise and feel the shock. The DT allows the controls to remain on longer than usual. I can tell something's wrong because the DT looks puzzled. "The equipment is not working properly," he says to himself. "You should have been dead already." He finally gives up, and says, "That's it. Beats me. Evidently not supposed to happen. I'm done." He rolls me to the room where people are gathering for my wake. I see people as they come in, but they can't see me. They know I'm still alive, but they celebrate and console my family anyway. It seems like a great party. Cecil has spent a lot of money on two wakes, but I won't die.

This was all a dream, but it all seemed very real to me. In fact, having a lupus flare that almost killed me really did happen.

Part 2
Stories About Lupus Warriors Diagnosed During Pre-Teen and Teen Years

The American College of Rheumatology (ACR) estimates that about twenty percent of people with lupus developed the disease before twenty years of age; however it is rare for lupus to develop before age five.[14]

According to the ACR, "There is no cure for lupus, but proper treatment can help significantly. Lupus can be life-threatening, especially when it affects vital organs such as the heart, lungs, brain or kidneys. The goal of treatment is to stop the inflammation by suppressing the immune system, helping with symptoms, and protecting organs from permanent damage. Treating lupus requires close monitoring by a pediatric rheumatology team, which may include doctors (pediatric rheumatologists and other specialists), nurse practitioners, physician assistants, nurses, social workers, counselors, and physical and/or occupational therapists. They will partner with the family, schools and other community resources to provide a child or teen with the best care for preserving physical and psychological health."[15]

The ACR recommends that children and teens with lupus be encouraged to live as normal a life as possible and that going to school, playing with friends, exercising, having a healthy diet and continuing family activities are all important. "Treatment is different for each child; each child is unique, as is each treatment plan."[16]

"Lupus has many different symptoms, and it affects each person differently."[17] Scientists report that lupus symptoms may include abnormal blood clotting, anemia, butterfly-shaped rash across cheeks and nose, confusion, depression, extreme fatigue, extreme weakness, dizziness, fingers turning white and/ or blue when cold, frequent fevers with no cause, hallucinations, headaches, low white blood count, memory and thinking problems, pain in chest on deep breathing, repeated miscarriages, seizures (convulsions), skin rashes, sores in the mouth and nose, sun- or light-sensitivity, unexplained hair loss, swelling around the eyes, and swollen and achy ankles, feet, glands, hands, joints, legs, and muscles.

According to the Lupus Foundation of America, "Many of these symptoms occur in other illnesses. In fact, lupus is sometimes called 'the great imitator' because its symptoms are often like the symptoms of rheumatoid arthritis, blood disorders, fibromyalgia, diabetes, thyroid problems, Lyme disease, and a number of heart, lung, muscle, and bone diseases."[18]

Lupus Does Not Have Me

by Helena Fields

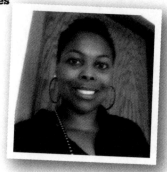

My journey with lupus began in the sixth grade when I first noticed this weird shaped rash on my face. Like many girls reaching puberty, I had a love-hate relationship with the mirror. I was always staring at myself and checking to see which features were appealing and which were not. Out of nowhere, here lay some kind of deformity that definitely would get me teased by all of the boys and some girls at school.

After a couple of weeks of its appearance on my face, I went to see my pediatrician. He seemed to just stare at my new facial attribute at first. Then he performed blood test after blood test but was still dumbfounded. I'm not sure if I had any other symptoms during this time. My mind was fixated on this winged abnormality stamped across my face.

After many pints of blood were drained from my body for testing and still no answers, the doctor decided it would be best to do a skin graft. I wasn't ecstatic about him slicing off a piece of my face, but I wanted to know the origin of this aberration. I was slightly relieved when my doctor wanted to send me to a dermatologist to have the skin graft. I was afraid he might not do a good job because he was quite old. I did not want to wind up with jagged features like a jack-o-lantern.

I should probably interject here by saying that it took almost three years from the initial appearance of the rash until I finally saw a dermatologist. The dermatologist looked at the rash on my face and then told me that he did not need to do a skin graft. He scribbled some notes on my chart and referred me back to my pediatrician. He said he would call him and let him know what it was. I wanted to scream, *Tell **me**! I want to know! Don't I get to know? It's **my** ****ing face!* But my mom and I followed his directions like good little patients often do and we left.

After a series of more blood and urine collections and over the course of an additional two years, I was finally referred to a rheumatologist. I would like to blame this delay on having an HMO. But hey, what do I know? The rheumatologist had already looked over all of my lab tests and patient history when he came into the room and simply said, "You have lupus." I thought to my-self, *What the hell is that?* He didn't really explain it much. He just wanted more of my blood and gave me a prescription. For what? I'm unsure. All I remember is after he named it, it changed me—physically, mentally, and spiritually. Lupus became a determin-ing factor in my life.

I would like to note that this whole process and diagnosis was pre-Google. My mom was even more clueless than I. That is probably the reason why she seemed to think that somehow, someway, I had contracted lupus from having sex, even though when my symptoms began, I was still a virgin.

By the time I was given my fate, the rash had already disap-peared. However, I now had experienced dramatic weight loss (which wasn't a bad thing since I had been overweight), thinning

"I went from being an A-student participating in extracurricular activities to barely going to school because of the external and internal pain. I felt like I had no control over my body. I didn't feel like me."

hair, and sore, swollen hands and feet. I also experienced a lot of mood swings and fatigue, which everyone dismissed as part of my teenage rebellion. Secretly, I drowned my sorrows with Mad Dog 20/20 and Boone's Farm wines while often contemplating suicide.I felt like a human test dummy. I was on various medications, and they didn't seem to help. I just wanted to die. I went from being an A-student participating in extracurricular activities to barely going to school because of the external and internal pain. I felt like I had no control over my body. I didn't feel like me. Even now when I go through a flare, my biggest issue is that I tend to dissociate from myself. I feel like I'm watching someone else go through the pain, so I just lie around and wait. I wait until the me I'm watching recovers.

I didn't really embrace managing my lupus or yearn to be healthy until I became pregnant with my son. Wanting to be a good mother coincided with my needing to be a better patient. For the first time in my life, I took my meds exactly as they were prescribed. I was on 10 mg of prednisone and 400 mg of Plaquenil (hydroxychloroquine) daily, along with a prenatal vitamin. I was very high-risk because of the lupus and other gynecological issues. I only had a small part of my cervix, and I wasn't expected to be able to carry a baby to full term. However, my six-pound baby was delivered via cesarean at thirty-eight weeks. He is now a healthy and vibrant eight-year-old.

My faith, along with the love and devotion I have for my son, helps me to focus on what is positive in my life. I still become tired and frustrated when I exhibit symptoms, but I try not to be sad for too long. It's hard to talk to people about how I'm feeling because when you look fine on the outside, they don't understand that you are a mess on the inside.

I have attended lupus support group meetings. The meetings are helpful, but they are also emotionally taxing. A lot of times, the members use it as a venting session, and I respect that; however, I survive by focusing on what's going right in my life. It's hard for me to open up and discuss what is wrong.

Being involved in lupus events and outreach is what excites me most. I would love to be more involved, but my work schedule is quite hectic. I have a lot of projects that I am working on simultaneously, and I hope these projects will help someone cope while living with lupus. But first, I need to discover more coping techniques for myself. I've been living with lupus for more than twenty years, and I'm still learning to cope. However, I am more determined now than I have ever been to overcome the challenges of having lupus. I have lupus, but I will not let it have me.

My Time is Coming
(Time to Fly Like a Butterfly)

by Chenise G. Rias

I'm a thirty-five-year-old married mother of fifteen-year-old twins (one male and one female), and I HAVE LUPUS. What is lupus? Well it's an autoimmune disease where your body fights itself. You may ask, "OK, so what does that mean?" Let me tell you my story, and maybe it will help you understand better.

In 1995, when I was in high school, I started noticing dark spots on my skin. I was very active and became very tired. Time went by, and the spots worsened. Then what I now know is a butterfly-shaped rash appeared on my face. I had always had beautiful skin and wondered what was going on. So I went to the doctor, and he just gave me some cream. Time passed, and the cream failed to improve my skin condition. Also, my joints were hurting. OK, something wasn't right, so I went back to the doctor. He took some blood, and I waited. Finally, the doctors diagnosed me with lupus. Ugh! What does that mean? I guess since I was young, it was simply stated to me, "Your body will be weak, and it will be hard for you to get over being sick quickly. Take this prednisone and Plaquenil, and we'll monitor you." They never explained that my skin would get worse, my joints would ache really bad, and I would be in and out of the hospital because of pneumonia, fluid on my heart, and kidney biopsies. Oh boy, I was so young. What was I going to do?

During my senior year in high school, I couldn't walk down the hallways or up the stairs to get to my classes. So instead of being with my friends or participating in senior activities, I took classes at home. Boy, that really sucked. I complained to my doctors, so they put me on enough prednisone to pump me up so that I would be able to get through the end of senior year and graduate.

In 1996, I was ready to attend college downstate. But as soon as I arrived, the hot weather was so bad that I had a major lupus flare. I had to come home to be hospitalized because the hospital down there didn't know what to do for me. Well, so much for my dream of attending the University of Illinois. "Boy," I thought, "this lupus thing is something else when even the heat can cause a flare."

A significant amount of time went by. I stayed home and went to school, dated, and met my future husband. I was doing well, moved out, fell in love, and got married. I went to the doctor for a regular check-up and discovered that I was pregnant. Now I was panicking. They never told me about lupus and pregnancy. Would I be OK? Would the baby be OK? I was happy and scared at the same time. I was told by more than one doctor, "You can't have kids; you must abort." This couldn't be; I couldn't believe this. Being raised in a Christian-based home, I knew I couldn't abort.

I was three months pregnant when I found out I was carrying twins. I was also experiencing serious problems: diabetes, pre-eclampsia, and definitely a lupus flare. By my fifth month, I was put on total bed rest at the hospital. By my seventh month, my body couldn't take it anymore. I had to get these babies out, or

I wouldn't be around to raise them. On April 11, 1998, I gave birth to my son, who was 1 pound, 9 ounces, and my daughter, who was 1 pound, 4 ounces. Look at what I have, and to think the doctors told me, "No!"

"But it seemed like every year between 2007 and 2009, I ended up in the hospital a week before Thanksgiving and a week before Christmas. That was it. I decided that I couldn't let lupus control my life."

From 2000 until 2007, I was in and out of the hospital, mainly for pneumonia. But since I had children now, I had to fight. Then in April 2007, I experienced one of the worst times of my life. I was very fatigued and really couldn't breathe. *"OK,"* I thought, *"I've been through this, I'll get some prednisone and be OK."* At least, that's what I thought! When my condition worsened, I went to the emergency room. Yep! It was pneumonia again, but a more serious strain than usual. My kids' birthday was in four days, so I had to kick this and make it home for them. The doctors came in and said my body was not responding to the antibiotics. I needed to be sedated so they could do an exam to determine the exact strain. This was their approach in order to determine the appropriate treatment plan. OK. What choice did I have? They performed the test, and I was unconscious for two days. My family was scared and thought that was the end for me. In my subconscious state, I must have still had my kids in my head because I woke up and was responding well to the treatment. But then other things were happening. I was retaining fluid so fast, and I couldn't breathe because of the fluids. My kidneys were to blame. So yes, on my kids' birthday, I started hemodialysis. Then to top it off, my doctors discovered that the heart murmur they were hearing was my mitral valve. Two days later, I had open-heart surgery to replace my mitral valve. My, my what was going on? I was only twenty-nine years old and going through all of this. But I fought and fought, regained my strength, and eventually came home. But it seemed like every year between 2007 and 2009, I ended up in the hospital a week before Thanksgiving and a week before Christmas. That was it. I decided that I couldn't let lupus control my life.

It's now 2014, and I haven't been hospitalized with any lupus flares since 2009. I've since been determined to control lupus and not let lupus control me. I'm working, still happily married, and raising two beautiful teens. Yes, I'm still on dialysis three days a week. However, I'm on the donor list. My time is coming. I will hold my head up and fly high like a butterfly!

A Strong Family

(Sisters & Lupus)

By Patricia L. Sanders

What a joyous occasion! This is our seventeenth family reunion. Man, we've come a long way. For the first Coleman reunion, held in 1967, we gathered in the back yard of my sister's house. This year, 1983, we've rented a banquet hall in the YWCA and have prepared a big buffet dinner. Today we are even electing officers. While the discussions are going on, I see my brother's son carry his teenage sister, Noel, into the room and place her body in a wheelchair. Her legs seem stuck in place and barely bendable, like those of an older person with severe arthritis. Though she smiles a lot and appears to have a pleasant and positive attitude, she looks very skinny and frail to me. Little did I know that within a few years, she would end up going through kidney failure, heart problems, and eventually, death.

Lupus was introduced to our family by my youngest sister, Noel. She presented in the doctor's office with a bad cold and a spider bite. Though I don't remember specifics, I know there were other symptoms that caused the doctors to suspect multiple sclerosis; then they suggested sickle cell anemia. My mom and sister told the doctors about other symptoms, which prompted them to run many tests. However, after learning more about the evaluation for autoimmune diseases, I now believe that many of the tests Noel received were "old-fashioned" and unnecessary.

My grandmother mentioned a cousin who had lupus. Also, doctors were discovering other parts of Noel's case that were puzzling. She was placed in the hospital for further testing and steroid therapy. There were complications from the different types of medicine given to her, affecting her kidneys and heart, before the doctors finally gave the correct diagnosis: lupus.

This was the beginning of Noel's senior year in high school. She had been very active in sports, and it was very difficult for me to see her in a wheelchair. Watching her being wheeled or carried around gave me an understanding of something my grandmother once told me: "You never know what life can bring your way. So you need to stay prayed-up, and keep Jesus close to you."

The hospital visits were hard on the family members, especially my mom. However, my family stayed prayerful and strong, and we were able to get through this phase of Noel's disease. While doing therapy, receiving dialysis, and having to be pushed around in a wheelchair, she continued going to school and completed the requirements for her high school diploma.

The whole family, including her brothers, sisters, and even her young nephew and niece helped to deal with her disease. They encouraged her to keep the faith, to believe there is no defeat in this family, and to believe that she *would* walk again. The time went by very quickly; she was walking with a walker, then a cane, then a brace. After she was back on her feet, she bought a car; it was a stick shift, I am proud to say. This act demonstrated her strength, determination, and willpower to do well in life. This also helped me to gain more faith in myself. The strength God gives to our family is truly what love is all about.

Somewhere along the way, I remember being told something about the same gene recurring among siblings every twelve years. The doctors speculated that since Noel and I were twelve years apart, I also carried the potential to have lupus. I'm not sure if this theory is true, but I was diagnosed with lupus and borderline diabetes in 2012.

Though my sister fought like a champion, she lost her battle with lupus in 1997 at the age of thirty-two. Watching her try to cope with lupus taught me many things. I deal with lupus by listening to my body, maintaining positive relationships with the medical community, staying active, eating right, getting plenty of rest, and taking time to meditate. I pray for a cure so that others can avoid the challenges of trying to deal with lupus.

Shaking Out the Cobwebs

by Lois Burleson

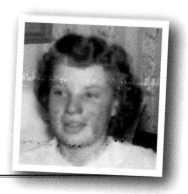

Lois says it's been a long time since she was diagnosed with lupus. She had to really search her memory, so she felt as though she was "shaking out the cobwebs" as she wrote her lupus story. This is her story.

It all began in the summer of 1951. I was the type of teenager who spent weekends at the beach developing a tan. This one weekend, the sunburn stayed. I didn't realize at the time I had the "typical butterfly rash." My doctor didn't want to touch the scabs that had developed. He didn't want to leave scars. He sent me to a dermatologist who took one look at me and said, "Lupus erythematosus."

I was treated at home with vinegar masks. Then the fever wouldn't go down, so I was put in the hospital. In the hospital, I was given ACTH (adrenocorticotropic hormone) intravenously for about three weeks. After being released from the hospital, I had to keep appointments with the dermatology clinic. Then I was hospitalized two more times and received the same ACTH treatments. I believe I was hospitalized about three weeks each time. I don't remember what meds I had to take at home, but it was probably cortisone. I continued my clinic visits, and then I was doing so well that I was able to stop the clinic visits. Then I was off all lupus medications for years.

I don't think lupus was involved, but, I need to mention that in 1954, I had a tumor in my neck. Doctors didn't remove it because then they'd have to replace it with a bone from another area of my body, I guess. Instead, the doctor performed a needle aspiration and determined it was not cancer. However, since the tumor had absorbed some of the bone in the vertebrae, I had to wear a surgical collar for a year until the bone re-calcified itself. All in all, I survived.

I married in 1955 and was advised to adopt children rather than bear my own. We adopted two children, one in 1959 and another in 1961. I was told that the longer I went without lupus symptoms, the better my chances for pregnancy. I gave birth in 1963 and 1967. I did not experience morning sickness and had very easy deliveries. I know I was not on any meds when I became pregnant.

It's only been recently that I was put on prednisone. I asked the doctor if it is the lupus. He said that it's polymyalgia rheumatica. Oh, well! I'm being weaned off the prednisone, and now I'm down to only 5 mg.

I had a partial right hip replacement in 2009, carpal tunnel in my right hand in 2013, and have aches and pains on occasion, but it's nothing serious. I'm still quite active. No one else in my family has any lupus symptoms. I'm one of a kind. Ha ha!

Part 3
Stories About Lupus Warriors Diagnosed During Young Adult Years

"Lupus is one of the cruelest, most mysterious diseases on earth. It strikes without warning, has unpredictable and sometimes fatal effects, lasts a lifetime, and has no known cure."[19]

L upus is unpredictable because it is a disease of flares (symptoms worsen and you feel ill) and remissions (symptoms improve and you feel better)."[20] Each case of lupus is different; symptoms can range from mild to severe and can come and go over time.[21] According to the Lupus Foundation of America, "Many of these symptoms occur in other illnesses. In fact, lupus is sometimes called 'the great imitator' because its symptoms are often like the symptoms of rheumatoid arthritis, blood disorders, fibromyalgia, diabetes, thyroid problems, Lyme disease, and a number of heart, lung, muscle, and bone diseases. Lupus patients may have various health effects, such as heart attacks, kidney failure, miscarriages, seizures, and strokes.[22] Though anyone at any time can be diagnosed with lupus, it is diagnosed most often between the ages of 15 and 44.[23] Ninety percent of lupus patients are adult females, however, children and males can also be diagnosed with lupus.[24] "Causes of lupus are unknown; scientists believe that hormones, genetics, and the environment are involved."[25] The Lupus Foundation of America says, "Today, physicians treat lupus using a wide variety of medicines, ranging in strength from mild to extremely strong. Prescribed medications will usually change during a person's lifetime with lupus. However, it can take months—sometimes years—before your health care team finds just the right combination of medicines to keep your lupus symptoms under control."[26] "With research advances and a better understanding of lupus, the prognosis for people with lupus today is far brighter than it was in the past. It is possible to have lupus and remain active and involved with life, family, and work."[27]

Since 1948, the U.S. Food and Drug Administration (FDA) has approved some medications for lupus, and these include:[28]

- Aspirin (FDA approved in 1948)
- Corticosteroids, including prednisone, prednisolone, methylprednisolone, and hydrocortisone (FDA approved in 1955)
- Antimalarials, such as hydroxychloroquine (Plaquenil) and chloroquine (FDA approved in 1955)
- The monoclonal antibody belimumab (Benlysta) (FDA approved in 2011)

Shining the Light on Lupus

by Ashley Chappell-Rice

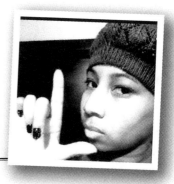

I was diagnosed with systemic lupus erythematosus (SLE) in 2012. Living with lupus is like the story of *Alice in Wonderland*. It is a very strange and unpredictable disease. If I explained to someone all the different symptoms and experiences I have suffered, it would sound weird, strange, and almost fabricated. One might wonder if I dreamed this all, especially since I look like an average twenty-six-year-old female. My weight is healthy, and I still smile, even after life gave me reasons to be sad. On the outside, I don't look sick at all. Lupus is deceptive that way.

I really showed symptoms of lupus long before I was diagnosed. Even as far back as my senior year in high school, my social life was affected by what I know now must have been lupus. I struggled with fatigue and could not seem to keep up with my friends and hang out for very long. At times, I had hair loss and skin rashes, but nothing seemed serious enough to consult a doctor. Lupus deceived me until 2012; lupus made its presence known that year, and my life has not been the same since.

One night, a nagging pain in my right arm interrupted my sleep. I couldn't get comfortable because my arm would not extend or bend. I continued to try to sleep through the pain, thinking it would go away. Yet the hours rolled by, and the nagging pain continued. Now it was time to go to work. As I attempted to get ready for work, I struggled to brush my teeth because my right elbow would not extend to turn on the faucet. I made a sad attempt at putting my hair in a bun. I tried to pull my pants up to my waist. I did the best I could to make myself presentable for work. I knew my appearance was sloppy, but I made my way to work anyhow.

It was early in my shift as a nurse, and we were very busy. As I rushed down a hallway, I slipped and fell, landing on the same elbow that was giving me problems. "Great," I thought, "it will only get worse." Even though I knew this elbow had given me problems prior to the fall, I now had an excuse for the problem and could blame the fall. I didn't know there were other problems lying dormant.

As life continued, I learned that I was pregnant with my second child. My husband and I were very excited, and I started to see an OB/GYN right away. Even though I continued to struggle with my right elbow, everything seemed fine for the first month of my pregnancy. I even learned how to get dressed without using the injured arm. This is the time when things became twisted. Remember, lupus is unpredictable and strange. It doesn't always have to make sense. One day while at work, my other arm started to have extreme pain to the point where I could not use it. I thought, "Now, I know I did not fall on this arm, and I cannot come up with an excuse or explanation for this. What's going on?" The limitation in the use of my arms became a big problem for my work performance. I was not able to complete my nursing tasks. A fellow co-worker suggested that I mention my concern for my arms to my OB/GYN. We were thinking it could be related to the pregnancy. "Great idea," I thought. I had never thought of that, and it would not hurt to mention it.

Sitting in my doctor's office, I began to explain my strange arm pains. As my doctor sat attentively listening, I began to realize I had several strange complaints. I explained that I had been short of breath and that my fingers had been turning blue occasionally. One time, while sitting in the pool outside under the sun, I became extremely fatigued and noticed rashes on my skin. I completely forgot about an important appointment. Taking a moment, the doctor says to me that I don't look good and that she thinks I have lupus. At first, I almost laughed, thinking that she was way off-base with that idea. I wondered, "What I could have said to make her suggest something so serious?" She told me she would do blood tests and that it would take about a week to get the results.

After I left the doctor's office, fear set in. What if I did have lupus? What would that mean? Before I had time to think this through, another twist on the roller coaster ride of lupus happened. Before we received the test results, my health aggressively became worse. My shoulders locked up, and I could not raise my arms. Shortness of breath became worse. Lying back in bed or a chair became painful with more pain accompanying every breath I took. The pain I had while breathing was unbearable; I sat up for three sleepless nights crying. I took Tylenol, but nothing worked. I knew something was very wrong and became concerned for my baby and myself.

Finally, I called my doctor to let her know how bad things had gotten. As I was explaining my new symptoms, she proceeded to tell me she just received my lab work. With my new symptoms and my positive ANA (antinuclear antibody) test, she was certain it was lupus. She wanted me to get to the hospital immediately.

I was admitted to the hospital. While waiting for my doctor, the hospital doctors and nurses attempted to make me comfortable by giving me various pain medications. Nothing worked. I had x-rays and CT scans of my lungs. I waited for my doctor's arrival in hopes that she could get to the bottom of my lung pain. When she arrived, she stated that she undoubtedly believed my symptoms and test results indicated that I have lupus. However, she wanted to be 100% sure, so she wrote an order for me to be evaluated by a rheumatologist. She went on to tell me that if I were diagnosed with lupus, my pregnancy would be considered high-risk; I would have to be seen by a specialist in rheumatology.

It took another day before I saw the rheumatologist. The pain in my lungs became so bad I wanted to stop breathing altogether. Finally, at about one o'clock in the morning, a nurse comes in and says that a rheumatologist called her over the phone, reviewed my medical record, and ordered a new pain medication for me. Desperate, I received prednisone intravenously. To my surprise, it helped some. Later that morning, the rheumatologist came to see me and dropped a bombshell. In his Russian accent and with an expression of pity, seriousness, and concern, he looks at me and says, "So Ashley, based on your complaints and lab work, it looks like you have SLE lupus." Honestly, at first, I felt a sense of relief. After trying different treatments for the pain and having nothing work, I was relieved to finally know what was wrong. The doctor looked puzzled. I guess that after seeing the relief on my face, he thought that I failed to understand how serious lupus could be, especially when the patient is pregnant. He explained more about my condition. Being pregnant caused my lupus to be even more serious. My lab results suggested I was in an extreme flare. My body could attack the baby. The lupus would probably be worse after pregnancy due to a rebound effect. Hearing this news scared me, but I knew he was only trying to prepare me for what I might have to endure.

I continued to take prednisone along with other medications for lupus. I stayed in the hospital for a few days under observation. During that time, my mind was flooded with many thoughts, and my heart was filled with lots of emotions. I was four months pregnant, was just diagnosed with a chronic severe disease, and was lying in a hospital bed suffering pain with every breath I took. My life had been completely turned around. I had to stop working immediately, and stress over bills would be added to other emotions I was having. I was in complete shock and afraid of the pregnancy's outcome. I was so overwhelmed.

After being released from the hospital, I followed up with the high-risk team at a teaching hospital. I was still not feeling all that well, but I had started to become accustomed to the pain. On my very first visit with the high-risk team, the doctor took one look at me and realized that I was a very sick person. She had me admitted right there on the spot.

While in the hospital, I saw a team of doctors. By now I had spent so much time suffering through exams, scans, blood draws, and interviews with doctors, I was starting to fear that I would spend my whole life in a hospital room. My husband stayed by my side, only leaving for work. Yet, I still felt alone. I knew of no one who was experiencing anything like this.

Once again I was released from the hospital, but I was short of breath even when lying in bed. I had an abnormally rapid heart rate, and my joints would lock up unexpectedly and for no reason at all. On top of it all, fear kept me from enjoying my pregnancy. Ultrasound results revealed there might be some issues with the baby. The doctors were still hopeful that even though the lupus was active, the pregnancy would be fine. This pregnancy was a roller coaster ride, and lupus was the conductor.

After seven months of pregnancy, things seemed to be leveling off. Nothing was getting worse; nothing was getting better. I began to feel that at least I was getting a baby out of all this bad news. I was adjusting to taking pills every day and having to be at home and off my feet. I decided to be positive. I stopped worrying. I was grateful for having a great doctor who was able to recognize the lupus right away. Despite the potentially devastating effects of a drug like prednisone, I was grateful that there was something to relieve the pain, at least to some extent.

Lupus is a random disease. It is unpredictable, and without warning, it can take a sharp turn for the worst. September 18, 2012, was a calm day for me. I did nothing much that day. I had hardly any pain and no new symptoms. My joints had good mobility. Although I had shortness of breath, the pain in my lungs seemed to be better. About 7:00 p.m., I sat on my bed waiting for my husband to return from work, when a sharp pain suddenly went down my belly. It caught me off guard. I tried to breathe and see if any other pain would occur. It could be a false contraction. I was not due for a while still. My five-year old daughter was home with me, and I didn't want to frighten her. I attempted to get my doctor's number so that I could call to let her know I was having pain in my stomach. While standing near the bed, my water broke, but only blood came. A pain took me to my knees, and I yelled out in agony.

"I woke up in the ICU, receiving blood transfusions and other IV treatments. I was bedridden and connected to several monitors. My family told me I was so swollen that I was unrecognizable. As I lay in the ICU, I felt that lupus had taken everything from me."

I called 911 and was rushed to a local emergency room. I was losing a lot of blood, and the ER doctors were trying to figure out what was wrong. It was getting hard to breathe. I was feeling weaker as I fought for my life. I heard the nurse yell out, "Should we call a code blue on her?" My blood pressure was 50/30. The nurses were struggling to get an IV started. As I was going in and out of consciousness, I remember one nurse placing a monitor over my stomach to get the baby's heartbeat. She turned the machine up loud. Then she shook me and said, "Do you hear that? That's your baby's heartbeat. Stay with us." I was trying to stay awake, but I felt no control over my body. I was rushed to the operating room and given fluid resuscitation, a temporary replacement for blood loss. I had suffered a placental abruption—my placenta had prematurely separated from my uterus, which I believed was due to the lupus flare. The only way to save my life was to do an emergency cesarean section.

I was given 200 mg of prednisone to get me through the surgery. It was so chaotic in that room before I went under anesthesia. As blood gushed from my body, doctors and nurses made a desperate attempt to save my life as well as the life of my baby. They were yelling orders across the room. They were making a special effort to keep me conscious. They were pulling my clothes off to prep me for surgery. They yanked me from one table to the next. I laid there helpless; I only had faith to rely on. The last thing I remember thinking was, I am going to die, but my baby will live because at least he has a heartbeat.

When I woke up, the environment was completely different. It was quiet—horrifyingly quiet. I realized I was alive; I had survived, but I heard nothing—no baby crying. I asked the nurse who was pushing me into recovery, "Where is my baby?" She could not speak. I said, "You have to tell me something."

She shook her head. "He didn't make it."

I began to cry. I didn't get a second of grief before my body began to hemorrhage again, and I lost more blood. I was in crisis yet again. The doctors began pressing on my C-section incision to try to control the bleeding. It was so painful. I just wanted them to get off of me. This time, I did not feel like fighting; I blacked out altogether. I woke up in the ICU, receiving blood transfusions and other IV treatments. I was bedridden and connected to several monitors. My family told me I was so swollen that I was unrecognizable. As I lay in the ICU, I felt that lupus had taken everything from me.

It was a long recovery process. It took a week in ICU and an additional week in the hospital before I was released. It was another year before the C-section healed. Just like the doctor had warned me, my lupus was worse. Gone were the days when I lived with no symptoms.

I tell these stories of how I was diagnosed and when I very traumatically lost my son to show that living with a chronic illness like lupus has no pause button. It continues every day, despite what one might have going on in life. It does not stop for marriages, birthdays, funerals, school, or financial problems. Sometimes the pain is so random. Sometimes I wake up, and my hands hurt so bad that it's hard to move them. The next day it might be my knees. Fatigue can keep me in my bed for two days. Muscle weakness might cause me to not be able to use a plate without dropping it. Most recently, I woke up one morning and could not walk at all. Housework is overwhelming, and sometimes the thought of eating just makes me nauseated. The sun makes me feel as if I have been drugged with Benadryl. The skin rashes are embarrassing and very itchy. My lymph nodes swell to the point that it is hard for me to swallow. My hair is falling out. Even though I look twenty-six, I feel seventy everyday. I don't remember what normal feels like. Each day is a struggle. I have to be aware of what I do and how I use my energy because I get exhausted easily. I don't have many friends because no one can relate to me or understand why I have to stay home.

To be honest, these symptoms I deal with daily are very annoying. It is sad to say that dealing with the symptoms has become my norm. I have learned to live with it. I make it around the symptoms because I believe that God kept me alive for a reason. I really focus on the one thing I can control, which is my thoughts. I make a choice to stay happy, grateful, and humble. My experiences with lupus were traumatic, but I decided not to let lupus win. I have decided not to quit. I am already in pain and hurting; I might as well get a reward from it by being a blessing to others.

I want to bring awareness to lupus because with awareness comes money for research for better drugs. America has had six iPhones invented in the last seven years or so but only one lupus drug in the last fifty years. Also, the mass public has little understanding of lupus and how people are suffering and even dying from this disease. There are people who judge me as lazy. They don't understand that I am sick, regardless of how I look. People with the obvious symptoms of lupus do not go to the doctors because they are unaware. I am grateful for this opportunity to tell my story in hopes it will **shine light on lupus.**

My Lupus, My Faith, My Story

(Living with a Debilitating Disease)

by Kelley Rose

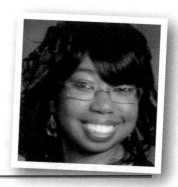

My health seemed to be in good shape when I was a college freshman in 2001. However, during my second year of college, I began to have joint pain that would become more intense as the weather changed to cold temperatures. I believe that every time I was stressing over things such as classes, exams, my long-distance relationship, and other cares of life, my arthritis pains would come upon me with a vengeance. The pain would begin in the evening right before bed. Tylenol seemed to provide some relief, but I could barely get out of bed the next morning. It was like my body was in so much pain that it stiffened up overnight. Some nights my sleep would be interrupted with chest pains and shortness of breath. The pain was so intense that I would pray and ask God to ease it. Then I would just cry myself to sleep. My mom would be praying for me too. We both just didn't know why I was in so much pain.

In 2002, I saw a rheumatologist and was evaluated for lupus. However, at the time, my doctors determined that a lupus diagnosis was not definite. So they just prescribed prednisone and calcium. My system did not tolerate those meds well, and I became sicker. I kept taking pain pill after pain pill, such as high doses of Tylenol or ibuprofen; whatever I could take to ease the pain. Nothing seemed to help. I continued working and at-

"When I heard the diagnosis, I had so many mixed feelings. I was relieved to finally know why I was in so much pain, yet I was curious to know what lupus is about. Also, it scared me because I felt that having lupus was going to affect my life in so many ways."

tending my classes. It was becoming more difficult for me to concentrate on my studies, but I was determined to continue my education. The only thing that my doctor had diagnosed me with at the time was rheumatoid arthritis (RA).

During the latter part of my sophomore year, I was barely making it to classes. Most of the time I just stayed in my dorm room trying to study, relax, and keep the pain under control. I stayed cold most of the time, and I always had a poor appetite. I would stress a lot, and that kept causing me to have more pain. Finally, I went to see another doctor, and he completed another evaluation for lupus. My brother took me to my follow-up appointment with my rheumatologist. The doctor told me that the test results, the description of symptoms, and my medical history showed that I have systemic lupus erythematosus (SLE). He asked me if I had ever heard of it before, and I said, "No." He briefly explained to me what the disease is, and then he prescribed two medicines called Imuran and Plaquenil.

When I heard the diagnosis, I had so many mixed feelings. I was relieved to finally know why I was in so much pain, yet I was curious to know what lupus is about. Also, it scared me because I felt that having lupus was going to affect my life in so many ways. The prognosis did not sound great, and no hope was in sight. Most days I would say to myself, "I will be just fine as soon as I get these flare-ups under control." I decided to go on with my college classes even though I continued to have aches and pains. It sounded easy, but in reality, it wasn't going to be an easy task.

Then in 2004, my husband and I got married, secretly. I was in my junior year of college, and he was in his senior year. I would travel to spend the weekends with him. It was rough traveling because I was still having severe joint pains. After my husband graduated, he began his grad school classes while I was still in my senior year. We finally told our parents and families that we were married. It was stressful for me because once I was married, I was no longer eligible for my parents' health insurance. That's when my stress really began to elevate, especially since I was just recently diagnosed with SLE. Also, my mom told me that since I was a married woman, my husband and I needed to find an apartment and live together. This caused even more stress for me. I was in my last year of college and trying to work full-time. My husband was not working then because he was in graduate school full-time. Things were not looking good at all for me.

My husband and I finally got our apartment together. I was paying all the bills because I was the only one working at the time. Since I was no longer under my mother's health insurance, I had to get a public-aid type of insurance. I was paying out of pocket for expensive health insurance that really was not helping me at all. But through it all, I continued to push through the aches and pains caused by the lupus. I just kept popping pain pills. God has truly been good to me in spite of my wrongs and my health condition.

In 2005, I noticed that I had some swelling in my hands, face, and feet. I didn't really worry too much about it because I thought it was just the lupus flaring up. I eventually went to see my rheumatologist, and she told me that I was retaining fluid. The fluid retention was causing my blood pressure to be elevated. So she prescribed Lasix (a diuretic) and blood pressure meds. Weight-gain caused by fluid retention and the pain from the lupus flares made it very difficult for me to move or walk. I had to buy bigger clothes and began to feel unattractive and very frustrated. My mom took me to a lupus support group, but as I was sitting there, I kept thinking to myself, *"These people are senior citizens. What am I doing here? I can't have lupus because this disease is for old people, not a young person like me."* I was in total denial. I decided I didn't want to go back to another support group.

Then one day I was talking with one of my former teachers. I shared with her that I was diagnosed with lupus, and she told me to apply for the Lupus Foundation scholarship. After submitting the application, I was granted the 2005 lupus scholarship. I felt so elated and more encouraged to keep on striving to achieve my goals.The spring and summer of 2006 was a very busy time for me, with more stress and lupus flares included. My husband and I bought a new house in April. In the same month, I was scheduled to graduate from college with my bachelor's degree. I was really not done with my teacher's certification program, but my health was beginning to get worse, and it was becoming harder each day to make it to class. I spoke with my academic advisor and told him about my health condition. He informed me that I had enough credits to graduate; I just would not be certified to teach. I was actually okay with that decision. I was so happy to be able to attain my goal of graduating from college.

After graduation, I started making plans to start my home day-care business. I became licensed and began to advertise. Then I received another piece of discouraging news about my health. My doctor informed me that my kidneys were shutting down. My creatinine levels were very high, which meant my kidney function was low. I began seeing a nephrologist (kidney specialist), and I was told that my lupus was being so aggressive and active in my body that it was attacking my kidneys. I was so sad that I wanted to cry. I wanted to give up on life. I was just beginning to handle the lupus pains, and now I was going into permanent renal failure. I spent most of my summer in and out of the hospital. While I was in the hospital, my doctor informed us that I should not get pregnant because of all my health issues; a pregnancy could put my life in danger. It was very hard for me and my husband, as newlyweds, to accept that. I was in denial of that too! The doctors continued to give me new medicines, and I began to take an infusion treatment called Cytoxan, a type of chemotherapy, to try and prevent my kidneys from totally shutting down. But I began to get sicker with the Cytoxan infusion. My hair fell out. The treatments eventually did not work. The lupus became more aggressive.

On September 7, 2007, I woke up so swollen and short of breath that I thought I was going to die. So my husband called the ambulance, and they rushed me to the hospital. When I got to the hospital, I was immediately given oxygen to help me breathe and some pain medicine because I had chest pain too. After they ran some tests, the doctor came in and broke the news. He told me that my kidneys had shut down completely and that I needed to have a catheter inserted in my groin in order to start dialysis right away before the fluid continued to build up around my heart. He told us that if that happened, I could die.

I was so mentally and physically tired of being in pain and going in and out of the hospital. Again, I was just ready to give up. But my mother's prayers and faith in God helped me to realize that I just needed to continue to trust in the Lord; that He will heal my body.

My first dialysis treatment was very rough and painful. But over the past six years of being on dialysis, I am getting better day-by-day. I had surgery in 2008 to create a dialysis fistula—an access point for my dialysis—in my left arm. Now in order to prevent blood clots and malfunction, my fistula has to be evaluated every three months.

I am managing my lupus by taking 10 mg of prednisone daily. I go to my dialysis treatments three times a week. On my non-dialysis days I often substitute teach at various elementary schools in my district. It's kind of weird, but since I have been on dialysis now for six years, I have fewer flare-ups that cause joint pain. I have to deal with kidney disease daily, and my focus is on how to live with lupus everyday. From time to time, especially in the winter, I may experience some arthritis pain. Usually I just take a Tylenol, and the pain goes away by the next day. As I move around during the day, the joint pain seems to subside but returns in the evening when the temperatures drops. I have developed anemia. Also, I suffer from loss of appetite; my rheumatologist says that is also associated with lupus.

In February 2009, my husband and I received our first foster son. We were so happy and thankful that the Lord had finally blessed us with the child that we always wanted.

Then in January 2010, I began having some pain on the right side of my lower back. I told my nephrologist, and he ordered an ultrasound to be done of my liver. As the tech was doing the ultrasound, she said, "Well I see nothing wrong with your liver, but I do see a baby down there." I didn't believe her, so she showed me on the monitor. She said that the baby was not a first trimester baby; it was almost a five- or six-month baby. I was so happy and scared at the same time—scared because I remembered the doctor had told me that I should not get pregnant because it could put my life in danger.

So after that appointment, I immediately called my husband at work and I told him that I was pregnant. I could hear the excitement in his voice over the phone. Then I went to my mom's house and asked her to come with me to my OB/GYN appointment. I was just supposed to be going to have my annual Pap smear, but when I told my doctor that I was pregnant, she immediately put me on a monitor to hear the baby's heartbeat. Then she told me to go straight to the hospital because I was now considered a high-risk pregnancy. My mother took me to the hospital, and when we arrived, the staff ushered me to the maternity ward immediately. They did an ultrasound and hooked me up to the heart monitors. The high-risk OB/GYN doctor came in to talk with us and to check my cervix. He told me that I was about seven months pregnant. I was so amazed because I didn't know I was pregnant all these months. I guess that was the reason I kept vomiting everything I ate. The doctor suggested having a C-section at first, but then he said that since I was feeling fine and my heart rate and blood pressure were normal, we would proceed with plans for natural childbirth. So I was admitted into the hospital and prescribed complete bed rest. I still had to have dialysis daily while I was in the hospital. I stayed in the hospital so they could closely monitor me and the baby.

Various tests revealed problems. My amniotic fluid level was very low; so it was very difficult to see the organs clearly. However, the doctors did determine that the baby was very underdeveloped and had no bladder. I was beginning to feel sad and scared. But then the doctor came and told me the worst news that any pregnant mother could hear: once the baby was born, he would most likely not survive very long because he was so underdeveloped and small. I was so hurt, mad, and disappointed. But the doctor kept telling me, "Guard your heart." At the time I didn't understand what he meant, but as time went on, I began to realize why he kept telling me and my family that.

I spent about three weeks in the hospital, and then the doctor said that I could go home. I knew I wasn't ready to go home yet because I would be busy doing things around the house and taking care of my 1-year-old foster son. My mom convinced me to stay with her at her house, so I would have help and could get more rest. Also, I was advised that I needed to have dialysis five days a week because the baby was making my kidneys work harder.

The morning of February 18, 2010, I woke up with severe

cramps. My mom realized I was in labor and started to time my contractions. We called the doctor who advised us to go to the hospital. The whole car ride to the hospital was painful because I could feel every bump. I had never been to a birthing class. I wasn't sure what to expect or what to do, so I just took deep slow breaths during each contraction.

Once we got to the hospital, they checked my cervix to see how far I had dilated. Then they put me in a birthing room. My mom called my husband at work, and he rushed to the hospital. After the anesthesiologist gave me an epidural, I slept for a while. Then a few hours later I woke up with a sharp pain in my side again. All of a sudden, the nurse came in to check my cervix, and she immediately called the doctors and delivery team. All I could hear them say was, "Show time." I was just waiting for the instruction to push. When I heard them say, "Push," I pushed maybe three or four good times. Then the baby was out. The doctor yelled, "It's a boy!" I was so happy that I had finally had a baby of my own. I was also scared because I didn't know if my baby was alive or not. I did hear his little faint cry before they hooked him up to a machine and took him down the hall to the neonatal intensive care unit (NICU). I was so tired, but I used what little energy I had left to pray for my baby to survive.

The doctors said he weighed 3 pounds, 10 ounces, and he was 15 1/2 inches long. The baby was named after my husband. Since my husband is a junior, our son would be the third generation, so we nicknamed him Trey. The doctor discharged me from the hospital two days after the birth, but Trey needed more time in the hospital. It was hard for me to go home without my baby. I wished I could stay right by his bedside to make sure he was OK.

I continued to go to my dialysis treatments. Every day I would either call or go to the hospital to check on Trey in the NICU. Even though Trey had some severe health challenges, he was fighting for his life. Trey had underdeveloped lungs and kidneys. He was also doing neonatal dialysis every day. I actually felt somewhat of a connection with him because we were both on dialysis. But I also felt bad because I never would want my child, or any child, to go through dialysis.

On April 13, 2010, I received a call in the middle of the night from the doctor. The directive was to come to the hospital as soon as possible because Trey had taken a turn for the worse. My mother-in-law drove us to the hospital. The doctor and the nurses were trying to give him oxygen because his heart rate was dropping. The doctor told me that he had developed an infection and was not getting better. So as the doctor stopped the respirator, my husband, my mother-in-law, and I just sat there. We watched my baby boy just pass away in our arms. We cried and cried and cried. I just kept thinking to myself, "Why did this happen to me? What did I do to deserve all this hurt?" But as time passed, I realized that it was God's will that Trey went on to Heaven. Now my baby boy is not suffering anymore. I know I am going to see him again some day. He will forever be in my heart.

I felt empty on the inside because I felt like I was robbed of really enjoying the feeling of being pregnant. I began to beat myself up mentally because I also felt that if I had known that

I was pregnant earlier, then I would have taken better care of myself, and the medicines that I was taking would not have harmed the baby. I went into a deep depression. I was at the point where I was despondent, and I stopped taking my meds. I just went to dialysis, came back home, and then went back to bed. I did not want to talk to anybody. My mother again began to pray for me. She tried to make me see that I couldn't give up because I had another baby who needed my love. She also suggested that I see a counselor so that I could talk about my feelings. I did get better and started taking my medicines again. I also began taking better care of myself and my foster son.

Trying to stay positive and prayerful helped to place me on the road that would begin the healing of my hurting heart. Something else happened to help me through this painful period in my life. In September 2013, my husband and I received our second foster child, a baby girl. Now our family is complete! I am so thankful and grateful that God has blessed me with two beautiful and healthy children. My faith in God is what keeps me strong and encouraged. I don't know about tomorrow or what my future holds, but I know that God is in control of my life. I have just learned to take things one day at a time and to do what I can to take good care of myself and my two children.

As I thought about my health, I realized that no one in my family, that I am aware of, has lupus. I am the first known case in my family. Wow! I must be pretty special. Even though I didn't accomplish my goals of being a licensed elementary school teacher, I have still accomplished a lot of things in spite of my declining health. I attend my monthly lupus support group meetings whenever I can, and I try to educate those who don't know about lupus. I continue to go to my dialysis treatments every other day and keep hoping for a kidney transplant. However, if I don't receive a transplant, I have faith that God will heal my kidneys and that they will begin to work on their own again.

"I have just learned to take things one day at a time and to do what I can to take good care of myself and my two children."

There is a gospel song that I love to sing because it encourages me. It states: "I just can't give up now. I've come too far from where I started from. Nobody told me the road would be easy. I don't believe He brought me this far to leave me." I am still here by God's grace and His everlasting mercy. God gives me strength to provide for my children and to take care of myself.

With a lot of support from my family and friends, I am doing the best that I can to maintain my health. In my spare time I enjoy shopping, singing in women's choir at my church, and just spending time with my family, especially my mother. She is such a huge inspiration and a support in my life. I love her so much, and I appreciate everything she has done for me. I thank God for her sacrifice, wisdom, care, and most of all her prayers. God is just so good to me! My strength is increased when I remember to keep God's word hidden in my heart. That I CAN DO ALL THINGS THROUGH CHRIST JESUS, WHO STRENGTHENS ME! This is just a portion of my testimony of living with a debilitating disease.

Advocate for a Cure

by Erica M. Collins, PhD

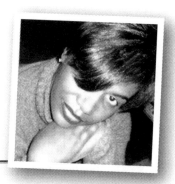

In September 2003, I entered the emergency room after experiencing numbness on the left side of my body from the waist down. I had three large lesions on my spinal cord and two on my brain. After spending ten days in the hospital, I was released with a diagnosis of multiple sclerosis (MS). Unfortunately, the medicine that was used to treat the MS caused me to suffer through temporary paralysis and two lengthy stays at a rehabilitation center. I experienced five hospitalizations between 2003 and late 2004 before finally receiving the final diagnosis: lupus. It took a little over a year for me to be diagnosed.

The doctors were confused because every time I had a relapse, the lesions on my spinal cord and brain showed no new activity. I often entered the hospital feeling bad and left feeling worse. After switching hospitals, I was eventually told I had systematic lupus erythematosus (SLE) that attacked my spinal cord. I began a four-year journey of intravenous and oral chemotherapy, large doses of prednisone, many hospitalizations, and several relapses of temporary paralysis. At times I would lose control of my bladder and the ability to walk.

In October 2008, I experienced a major setback. I lost control of my bladder and had temporary paralysis from the torso down.

After three days, doctors told me I had neuromyelitis optica with lupus antibodies.

Receiving this diagnosis caused me to aggressively seek alternative treatment. After a lengthy fight with my insurance company, I was finally approved for a stem cell transplant, which was completed successfully in December 2009.

The National Institutes of Health states that "neuromyelitis optica (NMO) is an uncommon disease syndrome of the central nervous system (CNS) that affects the optic nerves and spinal cord. Individuals with NMO develop optic neuritis, which causes pain in the eye and vision loss, and transverse myelitis, which causes weakness, numbness, and sometimes paralysis of the arms and legs, along with sensory disturbances and loss of bladder and bowel control."[29]

My medicine intake has been reduced from nineteen pills daily to six pills. I have been able to walk consistently without assistance, and I rarely suffer paralysis. Unfortunately, a dual diagnosis is not uncommon. The fact that I have lupus antibodies means that lupus is still lingering, and there is no cure for either diagnosis.

Day to day is always unknown for me, but what I have walked away with is the lesson that no one will fight for you harder than you do for yourself. Because my doctors didn't believe in stem cell treatment, I had to search for doctors who would consider taking my case and performing the procedures. They still say stem cell therapy is in its infancy, and they aren't convinced of its miracle capabilities long-term.

My family and friends have all been affected by my diagnosis. Many of them have had to make changes to accommodate me. They have to carry me for a while, but so far they haven't seemed to mind. They just all take on a role and carry it out for the duration. Our family members were already close; we became much closer. My sister and I are fourteen years apart, so I have always been a little bossy and more like a second mother. During this period I was forced to be more like a sister, and she became one of my immediate caretakers. I lost some friends, acquired some new ones, and gained a deeper bond with those I kept. I have had to learn not to be such an opinionated girlfriend because now I need my family and friends in a way that makes me humble. The things I took for granted are the blessings that I didn't realize I had.

I can see where the quality of life for others who didn't have access to better resources may have been affected. I can't say my life personally has been affected by the lack of public awareness because I have always been proactive and done my own research. Also, I sought the help of the Lupus Society of Illinois (LSI). I serve as the vice chair of LSI's Board of Directors, and that brings me a different kind of joy. I am most proud of my efforts to advocate for and raise awareness about lupus.

My disease is concentrated on my spinal cord, and there isn't a lot of public discussion about that type of lupus involvement. I worry a lot about waking up and not being able to feel my legs.

"I want the world to know that the continuity of health care is vital to quality of life. If you are diagnosed with lupus, be proactive in your care: read about it; sign up for lupus updates; think out of the box when considering treatment plans and doctors; make sure all of your doctors are aware of new research and updates...don't be afraid to call your doctors and ask if they are aware of a new article that you've found."

I continue to educate myself, and I remain proactive in my disease. I can tell you that there is more awareness about lupus now than when I was diagnosed.

I want the world to know that the continuity of health care is vital to quality of life. If you are diagnosed with lupus, be proactive in your care: read about it; sign up for lupus updates; think out of the box when considering treatment plans and doctors; make sure all of your doctors are aware of new research and updates...don't be afraid to call your doctors and ask if they are aware of a new article that you've found.

While we may not have a choice as it relates to our medical diagnosis, how we choose to look at life is within our control. Sometimes it takes a village to create change. So advocate on behalf of all people who have lupus, and a cure will come.

Angels Standing Guard

by H.L. Collins

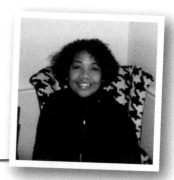

Sometimes life hardly seems fair. I don't think there's a single person who hasn't felt that way before. I doubt that I felt singled out by a greater power. Still something in me rejected all before me because it didn't feel quite fair or right.

As I stood there watching all the activities in the room, of which I was supposedly a participant, I didn't quite know my role. So when all heads were lowered, I bowed mine too. They then touched hands; I then touched too. When the priest began his prayer, I felt my body sway. So I bent my knees slightly and peered through one eye to stay balanced. I watched as the nurses, doctors and aides all bowed their heads in prayer, whispering words that I whispered too. These were prayers for my child and rejection of anything less than full recovery.

I can't remember all the words spoken during the short sermon, but I distinctly remember two things. As I stood trying heartily not to faint, not to change the focus of the activity, I tilted my head back casting my eyes upward seeking strength. I witnessed white-winged angels dancing above our heads. Now don't ask me if they were White, Black or of any color as they were faceless. But they danced with vigor, delight, and pure joy. I saw them clearly waving their arms and moving with a

> **"It is an insidious, life-threatening disease. It can cause you to watch the pendulum swing between life and death, good days and bad days, years of good health and years of bad health."**

powerful grace. Being in the presence of such images before this time, I recognized the significance of a band of angels. Yet this felt so different. It felt so different that a slight smile caught in the corners of my lips as I returned my attention just in time to hear, "Let thy will be done, on Earth as it is in Heaven."

The second thing distinct in my memory is the strong belief that this would be all right—a feeling of faith, a feeling of peacefulness, a feeling of gratitude. I looked down as my daughter, wrapped tightly in white bedding, rolled her eyes, then her head, backwards. She was totally aware of the moment and the omnipresence of the Lord and all the angels He had sent to her bedside. She then expressed a retiring smile so slight that it belied the fear she surely must have felt.

This was the day of her stem cell transplant. The day the Lord had giveth and could surely taketh away. This day had to have felt like a total reckoning between God and the devil in her own body. But it appeared to be a normal day to the others standing in attendance. It occurred to me this was a ritual they had all known and done before. Erica was the stranger and I the spectator; at least, that is how it felt.

Erica stands a full 6 feet, 3 inches in stocking feet. However, no one could know this, as she appeared so small and fragile in her hospital bed. Tears stuck in the corners of her glossy eyes, her mouth white and pasty taking short and shallow breaths while the smell of antiseptic permeated the room. But her brows were unfurled as she tried to mouth her own "Amen," joining the ritual while I stood resisting the urge. She, of all, appeared to feel the greatest content.

Lupus! It is such a devastating disease. Lupus wreaks havoc upon the friends and family of the chosen one. I won't use the word victim to describe people attacked by this devastating disease—these people are some of the strongest people I have ever known. Erica is no different. No different than any other person with lupus, but I am her mother. I did not choose this for my child; no mother would. We would choose to invite people to weddings, baby showers, graduations, and such. But then, as I said before, life isn't always fair—not to her, not to all the people who love her, and certainly not to people living with lupus.

So we continue to fight, continue to pray, and continue to get the word out that lupus wages sneak attacks upon us and our families when least expected. It is an insidious, life-threatening disease. It can cause you to watch the pendulum swing between life and death, good days and bad days, years of good health and years of bad health.

Erica made it through the stem cell transplant, but this fight is not over. It continues every day, every minute. The Lord sends angels to guard and keep us, always.

Kind of Like the Huxtables

by Brandi L. Collins

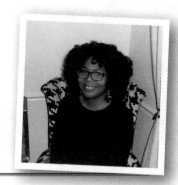

Ialways thought that my family was like the Huxtable family from *The Cosby Show*. Seriously, I was Rudy, though not nearly as precocious. My sister Semaj was cool and bohemian like Denise. My brother was a goofball but sort of charming like Theo. My dad was about as funny and sage-like as Cliff. My mom was elegant with the voice of reason, like Clair. We had a cousin who came to live with us, just like Pam. And we've even been known to break out into song and dance when the eggnog gets flowing during the holidays.

Then there was my sister Erica, the oldest sibling. Growing up she was the responsible-ish one, like Sondra, but also a social butterfly and mischievous, like Vanessa. She's fourteen years older than I am. For some reason she thought that made her my second mother and gave her leverage to boss me around. I, on the other hand, thought she was more like an annoying, underpaid babysitter—and made sure to push back every chance I got.

We also couldn't have been more different in personality. I was quiet and brooding; she was loud and a jokester. She was the one who always said what was on her mind—whether you wanted to hear it or not. I was the one who hid my true feelings behind sarcastic one-liners and quips. Needless to say the household dynamics often led to some comical, sitcom-like moments.

I have vivid memories of our humorous times together. Like the time she snuck out and took our parents' car for a joy-ride—with me in the backseat. Then there was the time—well . . . times—she threw a party when my parents were out of town, and put me in the room with a videocassette of *Dirty Dancing* and a pizza. Or the times when we stayed up all night laughing and drinking appletinis, or flirtinis, or whatever "-tinis" were popular at the time.

There are other less comical, but no less memorable, moments too—like the overwhelming pride we felt for each other when we graduated college, Erica from a PhD program and I from law school. There was the time I stood next to my sister as her maid of honor, bawling my eyes out as she got married. Then there was the time she supported and staunchly defended me to our parents when I whimsically decided to move across the ocean to London, England. Then there was the time I saw her lying in a hospital bed, more vulnerable than I could've ever imagined my six-foot-three-inch, loud, bold, and beautiful sister could ever be. I remember the time my dad silently cried as he shaved her head before she had to undergo a rigorous stem cell replacement, after what had been several rounds of useless chemotherapy. There was also the time I realized that she may not be by my side forever, bossing me around until the very end.

Before her diagnosis, my sister had been complaining of various ailments, such as joint pain and extreme fatigue. There were even less obvious symptoms that we would learn later were also part of it, headaches and sometimes disorientation. I wrote it off—she was running around too much, she had just moved back to Illinois from Texas. I thought maybe the stress of that had gotten to her. "She'll be OK," I thought to myself. That's the thing about lupus and other autoimmune diseases— the symptoms can be so subtle and unpredictable that you don't know what's happening. As a family member or someone watching from the outside, it's easy to be dismissive because the symptoms are often hard to see. I remember jokingly calling her a hypochondriac because it seemed like there was always something wrong. In hindsight, it was likely the disease manifesting itself over a longer period of time than any of us realized, but it didn't occur to me that they were all connected somehow.

Then I got the call. My big sister, the one that had always been there, taking care of me (even when I said I didn't want her there), had been taken to the emergency room.

She couldn't feel her legs, they said.

There were lesions on her spine, they said.

They had no idea what was wrong with her or how to stop it, they said.

This can't be real, I thought.

I guess that's why they call it a "mystery illness"—it's hard to diagnose, treat, or understand. As a family member standing by and watching helplessly, it's hard to quantify. How can you fight a monster that you can't even see? If the doctors don't even know what they're dealing with, how can we as family deal with it?

The thing about my sister is that she's never been the damsel-in-distress sort. Literally from her hospital room, she and Mom sat researching and poring over any information on the Internet they could find, to try to figure out what was happening to her body. They demanded tests that doctors normally don't automatically give. They asked pointed questions that patients usually don't know to ask.

Eventually, we got a diagnosis. Only then could we, and also the relentless team of doctors, choose the right weapons. Over a month later, Erica got out of the hospital. After physical therapy, she finally was able to put away the walker. Eventually, she slipped her four-inch heels back on, steadfastly marching towards the light at the end of the tunnel. And in true Erica fashion, she didn't just stop with her own recovery, she became active with the Lupus Society of Illinois (LSI). She's not just an active member, she is the vice chair of the Board of Directors. She's used every opportunity to share her story. That's just one reason why I love her so much—because she's a fighter and a natural born advocate, not just for herself, but for countless others.

I wish I could end the story there, but unlike *The Cosby Show*, this isn't a sitcom. Things don't get neatly tied up in a bow and resolved at the end of the half-hour. From the day she was admitted to hospital, this has become a never-ending journey—close to a decade and counting—with ups and downs that even the best screenwriters in Hollywood couldn't predict.

"That's the thing about lupus and other autoimmune diseases—the symptoms can be so subtle and unpredictable, that you don't know what's happening. As a family member or someone watching from the outside, it's easy to be dismissive because the symptoms are often hard to see. I remember jokingly calling her a hypochondriac ... In hindsight, it was likely the disease manifesting itself over a longer period of time than any of us realized, but it didn't occur to me that they were all connected somehow."

Honestly, I don't know what the hell else could happen, and that terrifies me. I just want her to be OK, and I want to protect her like she's protected me my whole life. But even as legions of researchers and doctors struggle to get a handle on this "mystery illness," there remains so much we don't know, and no known cure. The treatments available come with harrowing side effects.

As family members, we have to prepare as much as we can for the reality that these stories may not have happy endings. But every day, even when I don't always show it, I try to cherish and hold on to the beautiful moments that I've been given with my family, my sister. The laughter and the tears, I hold them all. And together we march forward, or maybe, like the Huxtables, we'll dance on.

Grateful for Life
(Establishment of a New Normal)

by Robinzina Bryant, retired FBI special agent

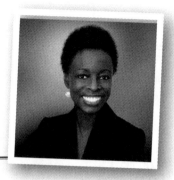

My initial symptoms of lupus arrived as unwelcome guests while I was serving my country as a special agent for the Federal Bureau of Investigation. They showed up, hung around, and then began to help themselves to my good health against my protest. I first experienced extreme fatigue, noticeable skin lesions primarily on my face and back, hair loss, and debilitating joint pain in my wrists, feet, and knees. With intention to preserve my health and my vanity, I addressed my symptoms vigorously with home remedies and visited a variety of health care professionals. And, oh how I prayed! I intuitively knew something was happening in my body that was beyond my ability to self-diagnose and treat.

It was my dermatologist who first suspected I might have lupus. After doing a biopsy of a rash in the center of my back, he referred me to a rheumatologist at one of the teaching hospitals in Chicago. His suspicions were confirmed. In April 2005, after six months of hopping from doctor to doctor who only treated the symptoms, I was finally diagnosed with lupus.

I was now armed with a diagnosis and a course of medication. I then began taking steps to arm myself with knowledge on how to live with and manage this incurable internal attack on my immune system. My older sister had been diagnosed with lupus five years earlier, and after a short course of treatment with the same meds I was prescribed, her lupus went into remission and has not returned to date. This caused me to be very hopeful about my prognosis.

Within three weeks I began to feel and see some positive results from the medications. My joint pain began to ease. Though many of my skin lesions cleared up, I continued to have a bright reddish butterfly-shaped facial rash distinctively associated with lupus. I was the lupus patient who drew the attention of all the medical students, fellows, and residents. They just had to have a look at me.

My special agent duties during this period included serving as the division recruiter. This responsibility required boundless energy, and, for all intents and purposes, made me the face of the bureau. My appearance in April was not fit to be a walking advertisement for anything, and at June's end, I took what I intended to be a two-week hiatus to rest. Two weeks later, after presenting with fever and unbearably painful, swollen hands and feet, I was hospitalized.

After a full blood work-up and testing of aspirated fluids from my hands and feet, it was determined that I had somehow contracted a methicillin-resistant Staphylococcus aureus (MRSA) bacterial infection. It had invaded my bloodstream by the time I arrived at the emergency room. I was informed that had I waited another forty-eight hours, I would have died. I actually had sought treatment at an ER near my home two days prior. Doctors in that ER, convinced I was suffering from gout, prescribed medication accordingly and sent me back home without ever having aspirated any fluid. When my pain continued and became intolerable, one of my sisters drove me to my familiar ER more than twenty-five miles away. I arrived with swollen fingers resembling bratwurst sausages. My usual size seven feet were so swollen that I had to borrow my next-door neighbor's shoes that were men's size eleven.

MRSA tried to kill me. It took me down to eighty-seven pounds and destroyed all the cartilage in both of my wrists and big toes. This teaching hospital conducted four hand surgeries that were designed to alleviate the swelling and allow drainage. I believe they were incision and drainage procedures. Using huge, fear-inducing syringes, the doctors aspirated my feet. Although the swelling in my feet subsided, the procedures left me with bunions and an imbalanced gait. I was limp-handed and unbalanced. From the looks of my scars, it was as if holes were drilled in my hands and wrists to allow the septic fluid to drain, but at least I was still alive.

When I was finally able to leave the hospital, I was required to go to the Rehabilitative Institute of Chicago (RIC) to regain strength as well as to learn how to do things with the limitations that limp wrists and the unbalanced gait imposed. The therapists at the RIC were amazing. They were tough on everyone, and they pushed until every muscle burned. Mentally, I drew strength from the physical training I had undergone at the FBI Academy. At the RIC, I remember crying and praying a lot but pushing through. I emerged from the RIC stronger, but was told by the teaching hospital that there was nothing more that could be done for my hands. I was scheduled for a visit to the Mayo Clinic for a second evaluation and advised that upon my return, I should consider double amputation of my hands and subsequent prosthetics. Instead, I sought out a new hospital immediately.

I got settled in at a different teaching hospital in January 2006 and met my new rheumatologist, and we clicked immediately. She was a woman of both faith and science, and I knew she would not only doctor me but pray for me as well. During her initial evaluation, she told me she wanted me to be seen by a particular orthopedic surgeon. Believing he would save me a trip to Mayo, she scheduled the appointment. She stoked my hope.

The new orthopedic surgeon took x-rays and thoroughly examined my hands, after which he stated with guarded optimism, "I think I can save your hands." Hope sprang up in me, and we began our journey of surgeries that would lead to being fitted for bi-lateral wrist implants, artificial joint replacements similar to knee and hip replacements.

My first surgery with this gifted surgeon went off without a hitch. Therefore, the following month, I confidently returned to the operating table for surgery number two. But this time, something went terribly wrong. While being prepped for surgery by the anesthesiologist, I had a seizure and then went into full cardiac arrest. My heart stopped. Cardiopulmonary resuscitation was performed for twenty minutes. I was shocked three times with the electronic paddles without any successful resuscitation. I was then packed with ice and put into a clinical state of hypothermia to hopefully preserve my cardiovascular and neurological stability and, of course, to bring me back to consciousness.

The surgeon told me later that I began to remove the icepacks myself—something of which I have no recollection. However, I am keenly aware that I do not like anything cold against my skin. Folks have often asked if I saw a bright white light while away for twenty minutes. I did not. But I believe it's equally, if not more, important that I did not see fire either. I trusted this surgeon and prepared to go back under the knife with him as soon as I was healthy enough to do so. However, for this surgery, I would have a different team of anesthesiologists. To date, I have had a total of twelve hand/wrist surgeries with this surgeon.

The six months following my cardiac arrest were emotionally tough for me. During this period of time, my surgeon told me that I would never again serve my country as an FBI agent. The damage to my hands and wrists from MRSA and the subsequent surgeries had resulted in my not being able to handle my weaponry. I had never defined myself by my profession, but the reality that it was over was emotionally devastating. As my surgeon delivered this news, I just sat in his office and cried. To my surprise, he cried with me, and in that moment, my surgeon became my friend.

I kept a journal throughout many years of my illness, especially during the worst times. I wrote in June 2006 that I was thinking a lot about going home and being with Jesus. I was not feeling depressed; rather, I was just emotionally and physically tired. Upon awaking from my cardiac arrest, I remembered that I did not have a will in place, so I made an appointment in June to get one along with powers of attorney. I also filed a do-not-resuscitate order with the hospital during this time. I wrote about the wonderful and full life I had lived. I wrote of how I had fulfilled just about every dream of mine, with the exception of getting married. I wrote of how I had fulfilled my educational goals and had an exciting and fulfilling career with the FBI. I wrote of the things I would miss, such as being able to see my twenty-one-year-old sister, whom I raised as my daughter when our mother died, as a fully mature adult; hanging out with my wonderful sisters; growing old with my closest girlfriends and seeing how we would be as old ladies; and seeing how my nieces, nephew, and god brother's children turned out. I wrote that although I would miss a few things, I was ready to die if death would welcome me. I did not do anything to hasten my death. I was not suicidal, and I would never do harm to myself. Instead, I prayed and asked God to simply not allow me to survive my next scheduled surgery on June 20, 2006.

Leading up to that date, I got my affairs in order and said what I hoped to be goodbyes to those I loved without defining them as such. In my prayer, I told the Lord that if He did not cooperate with my plans and I survived the surgery, I would take that as a sign that He had more work for me to do. I promised not to speak to Him any time soon about wanting to die.

My next journal entry began, "Still here!" I was surprisingly disappointed to have awakened from surgery.

In the fall of 2006, lupus began to attack my heart and kidneys. My heart was not pumping properly, and its chamber pressures

"The six months following my cardiac arrest were emotionally tough for me. During this period of time, my surgeon told me that I would never again serve my country as an FBI agent . . . As my surgeon delivered this news, I just sat in his office and cried. To my surprise, he cried with me, and in that moment, my surgeon became my friend."

were off-kilter. Additionally, my kidneys were beginning to fail. In November 2006, I was hospitalized and evaluated for heart and kidney transplants. Even though my health had taken a turn for the worse, I kept my promise to God and fought for my life through all the valleys that lay ahead of me. I arrived home in December, thankful that I did not need heart surgery as was initially anticipated. Instead the cardiologist performed a right heart catheterization and injected various medicines directly into my heart. In addition, he found some oral medicines that further stabilized the pressures in my heart's chambers, and that allowed my heart to pump normally again.

My lupus/MRSA-induced arthritis worsened throughout the end of 2006 and into 2007, and I seemed to stay in a lot of pain. My rheumatologist had scheduled a chemotherapy treatment for me on April 30, 2007, with hopes of it alleviating my arthritic pain and kick starting my kidneys into better functioning. It was not to be. My kidneys failed completely on April 29, and I had my first dialysis treatment. After completing my second treatment, I fainted. Dialysis was an adjustment for my 5-foot 3-inch 105-pound frame and an even bigger adjustment for my mind and spirit. This event broke me. My hope was shattered.

My first three weeks at the dialysis center were depressing. The dialysis center provided a living demonstration of how my life would progress for me if I did not receive a kidney transplant. Back in June when I asked to die, I wanted to go peacefully and quietly by just not waking up after surgery. At the dialysis center, I was forced to watch how my death would unfold as my body deteriorated from prolonged dialysis treatments. I watched people come into the center initially walking independently, then on walkers, then in wheelchairs, and lastly laid out on stretchers. Then I didn't see them anymore. I knew they had died. After getting through those first three weeks, I realized that I really did not want to die, and I did everything within my ability to stay as healthy physically, spiritually, and mentally as I could. I chose to live. I searched for reasons to live and soon began to view my dialysis machine as my lifeline which kept me present and connected with those I loved and cared about. I re-gathered my shattered hope.

I was physically incapacitated for periods between July 2006 and July 2009. Although my energy levels were impacted by lupus and the drain of dialysis, my body began to grow a bit stronger. I predictably and intermittently required naps. Starting in 2007, whenever I was able to tolerate it, I tried to get out of the house every now and then and re-engage with life and society. I had a wonderful team of friends, family, and former colleagues who played amazing roles in my coping process. Time does not allow me to share the incredible stories herein, but suffice it to say, I survived because members of my team were my life support system!

In 2008, I became a grandmother. When I watched my grandson come into this world, I was infused with a fresh hope to live and to watch his new life grow and develop. His presence was refreshing. I made a decision to create a mission for my life because I planned to live with a purpose. I determined that if dialysis or lupus took me out, that it would not happen for a very long time. I decided to dust off my law degree (a degree I had received before becoming an FBI agent) and to sit for the Illinois bar exam. I was already barred in Michigan, but had joined the FBI three years after becoming barred, so I had no reciprocity in Illinois. I needed to take a refresher bar review class, and it was very challenging getting this done while on dialysis.

Looking back, I know it was only the Lord that carried me through it all. I would attend dialysis, go home, take a nap, awaken, get a bite to eat, catch a commuter train to downtown Chicago, transfer to a bus, arrive at Kent Law School, and then sit for three or four hours in the bar review class. It was physically torturous. Upon passing the bar, I shopped my résumé and asked several attorneys to allow me to volunteer for free in order to reacquaint myself with the law. I knew I was interested in doing estate planning due to my own experience of nearly leaving earth without having my estate secured; however, I was open to doing just about anything except for criminal defense work. I landed with probate, an area of the law that fits very nicely with estate planning.

I volunteered on my non-dialysis days with set hours and did whatever my body allowed on my dialysis days. I volunteered around my surgeries and whatever hospitalizations (planned and unplanned) that arose. In 2009, I took a bold step. I incorporated and formed my own solo law practice. It has been quite a challenge, yet it has allowed me to manage my health-care needs.

In September 2011, after four and one-half years of dialysis, I received a call from a cousin informing me that she had undergone compatibility testing and had recently learned she was a match. I was grateful beyond expression, humbled by her selflessness, stunned and excited about the possibility of receiving a new kidney. My hope swelled. The following month, my cousin and I underwent a textbook-perfect kidney transplant. I made urine before I was even stitched up—so they tell me.

I am now two years post-transplant, and my lupus is cautiously managed and controlled. I try not to dwell on what lupus took from me, but rather I am grateful for being able to establish a new normal for myself. I am grateful for my journey of illness as it has expanded my capacity for empathy and has put life in sharper perspective. I am grateful for a second chance at life made possible by my selfless and brave cousin, willing to be my life-giver. I am grateful as well for all those individuals who prayed for me, encouraged me, supported me emotionally and financially, and loved me back to health. I am grateful for life.

Something Called Lupus

by Jocelyn O. Carreón

In 1980, I was a teenager working at a community medical clinic. Severe pain in my back and legs and dark spots on my face prompted me to see one of the doctors at the clinic. During the examination, I noticed that the doctor seemed puzzled. She asked me if I had fallen or if something had happened that might have caused injury to my back. She ordered blood work and an MRI. The MRI revealed that I had a herniated disk. The doctor said that I needed to see a back specialist. That was not a great option for me since I had little money and limited health insurance coverage.

> **"When lupus was mentioned to me in the 1980s, I thought I was having health problems because I was doing too much, working two jobs . . ."**

Then after reviewing the lab results, the doctor told me I had something called "lupus." I had no idea what that meant. She tried to explain what lupus was, but I did not understand and was not given any written material to study. I was scared, yet I did nothing. I didn't know about lupus or its potentially devastating effects. I didn't fully understand how important it was to attend to my condition. I felt I could just live with the pain, and I did so for the next five years.

The next time I heard this word "lupus" was around 1985 when the joint pain became really bad, and I was always tired. I saw a rheumatologist who said, "You have beginning rheumatoid arthritis, possible fibromyalgia, and borderline lupus." I was really confused, thinking, five years ago a doctor said I had lupus, and now this doctor is saying I'm borderline for lupus. This must not be too serious; maybe it's not important; maybe I'm getting better. The doctor didn't say anything about treating me or prescribing medication. Even though I still felt scared, uninformed, and confused about what was happening to my body, I failed to push for answers. I continued to see that doctor, however it seemed the only reason for making visits to the doctor was to get blood work done. I was afraid of needles, so that was another issue for me. That doctor treated me for two years by reviewing tests and x-rays; however he did nothing for the lupus. I didn't even think about asking about the lupus, uh borderline lupus. I just kept making office visits, getting painful and frightening blood work done, and just dealing with the fatigue and joint pain.

Then, my joint pain and swelling increased. Fatigue became so common I could barely function on my two jobs. The only answer from the doctor was, "You're too young to be in this much pain and to be this tired!"

I told him, "What does age have to do with how I'm telling you I feel?"

I started asking the doctor for a more complete explanation about my condition. He seemed disgusted with me for asking questions. I think maybe he was frustrated for two reasons: he couldn't determine a definite diagnosis and I was not just accepting what he said without a full explanation. Finally, he decided to order more blood work. When I saw the doctor again, he informed me that he had reviewed the lab results and that I needed to have my eyes examined.

I said, "My eyes?" He shook his head in apparent frustration and anger. Then, he said, "Calm down. I want this exam because it needs to be done before I can put you on a medication." The thought of a medication affecting my sight scared me. I wanted to know what kind of medication was this that could affect my eyes. He told me it was called Plaquenil. But he never told me that it is used to treat lupus! Now as I think back, I regret not following up, but limited financial resources and not being able to get answers were roadblocks for me. Plus, I thought all rheumatologists were alike, and I didn't know where else to go. I didn't know anyone else who had the disease. I had no one to help me understand.

> **"Even though I still felt scared, uninformed, and confused about what was happening to my body, I failed to push for answers."**

When lupus was mentioned to me in the 1980s, I thought I was having health problems because I was doing too much, working two jobs. If the doctor had said it was to treat lupus, I would have taken the Plaquenil. But I was not going to take something without knowing why I was taking it. So, I did not take the Plaquenil in the '80s, and I didn't see that doctor anymore.

I just continued to suffer until 1988 when I had a stroke that left me partially paralyzed for almost three weeks. During the same time, there were issues with my heart. The cardiologists said something was causing too much stress on my heart and that's all they knew. Too many things were going on, and I needed some answers. My mother suggested that I try to get help at a teaching hospital.

In 1990, I contacted the University of Chicago Medical Center (UCMC) and discussed my health issues. I never thought about mentioning the previous borderline lupus diagnosis, so UCMC scheduled my appointment with their endocrinology department. After the endocrinologist examined me, discovered all the swelling, and heard about the pain in my joints and neck, he ordered blood work. He told me my test results showed that my body was producing too much insulin and I was about to go to an extreme limit in my body. They further indicated that when my body reached that extreme limit of insulin, it would respond like that of a full-blown diabetic. However, it would not be the same as type 1 or type 2 diabetes, even though doctors will diagnose it that way. I also found out that I was producing more testosterone than estrogen, and I was diagnosed with polycystic ovary syndrome. I started to develop brittle facial hair like males have. Thanks a lot! The doctor seemed to be most concerned about the polycystic ovaries. He prescribed injections and placed me in a study group with other women who had even more facial hair than I did. I still saw my local primary doctor while I was in the study at UCMC.

Then in 1994, I was diagnosed with goiters and nodules on the left side of my thyroid. My uvula (small bit of flesh dangling down in the back of the throat) and tonsils were also enlarged. In 1995, I had the first surgery on my thyroid gland and uvuloplasty (surgery to remove the uvula) at a hospital near my home. I recovered from the surgeries, and even though I suffered with fatigue, I finally returned to my two jobs. Things stayed the same until about a year later.

One day in 1996, I woke up with a head as big as a sumo wrestler! I went straight to the endocrinologist's office. Didn't pass go; didn't collect $200. I wanted the doctor to see me immediately.

After completing laboratory tests, doing CT scans, and attempting a biopsy of my thyroid, the doctor said that there were goiters for sure, but they were so hard he couldn't complete a successful needle biopsy. I was told that something was pushing my trachea out of alignment, risking my life, so I was scheduled for another thyroid surgery. As they began the surgery, cutting through scar tissue, they discovered papillary cancer. I was in surgery for fourteen hours. Then I was on life support in the intensive care unit for days. But God woke me up out of a coma. I didn't know where I was or how long I had been there. I couldn't talk, and my blood pressure was extremely high. After getting my blood pressure under control, I was released from the hospital and started radiation treatments.

More things were happening. I lost my hair and eyebrows. I had been diagnosed with epilepsy around age nineteen; the seizures started occurring again. I lost most of my teeth. Then I had a heart attack.

I can't remember the exact dates, but I know I filed for Social Security Disability three times and was denied each time. Assumptions had been made and notes had been written indicating that I probably smoked cigarettes, was an alcoholic, and abused drugs. I retained an attorney, had my day in court, and the truth was revealed. Finally in 1997, after about three years from my initial filing date, I was awarded full disability benefits.

Then the predicted diabetes-like diagnosis came. I was on my way home from a church service one Tuesday night in 2002. Halfway home, I experienced muscle and joint cramps from hell. I had to pull the car over to a parking lot. My foot had turned sideways from the muscle spasm. After a while, I was finally able to get home. The next morning, I drove myself to the emergency room. At first, my glucose registered around 200 mg/dL. But when laboratory tests were done, my glucose level registered over 600 mg/dL. Then four doctors came into the cubicle. I felt like I was in the circus. One doctor said, "You are a miracle to be alive. We have never heard of anyone having a glucose level over 600 and functioning!"

I registered as a diabetic just as doctors at UCMC had predicted in 1990. This lasted until 2010, for eight years. Then it stopped completely. I am no longer considered a diabetic.

About three years ago, I saw my primary doctor because I was having even more joint pain. This time, I mentioned the long ago borderline lupus diagnosis. My primary referred me to a rheumatologist who did blood work, reviewed my symptoms, and gave me a definite diagnosis of lupus. I've been on Plaquenil since then. At one point they also prescribed prednisone, but it made me sick, so I told my doctor I didn't want to take it. I also take other medications for all my different health issues.

I still have to deal with various health issues. I have diverticulosis (small pockets in the wall of the digestive tract), two livers, an enlarged heart, acid reflux, potassium deficiency, sleep apnea, polycystic ovary syndrome, carpal tunnel, rheumatoid arthritis, and epilepsy. During a lupus flare, I might experience headaches, joint pain, foot pain, gout, nausea, swelling of hands, inability to taste, daily hair loss, and irritable bowel syndrome. Now the lupus is attacking my kidneys. Tests show that my kidneys are functioning at only twenty percent, so my doctor has ordered a biopsy.

There are things I can't remember, but I know I went many years when nothing was done to treat my lupus. I feel that many medical problems I suffered over the years were lupus-related, but that possibility was not always considered. Not knowing about lupus and what it could do to the body caused me a lot of pain and suffering. I feel like I've been alone in the struggle - that I've always had to fight to get answers to questions concerning my health issues.

I am still haunted by the lack of lupus awareness within the general population and especially within the healthcare community. Good doctors are so critical to those of us with lupus.

I feel that I would not be as damaged if I had pressed to get help at places that did more research. I am grateful to rheumatologists who really know about lupus, those who put forth the extra effort to learn about lupus, and those who conduct activities that promote discovery of new information. I am grateful that I'm still here, especially after doctors warned me on three different occasions that I wouldn't survive. I am grateful that I survived in spite of all my challenges. I'm still alive. Thank God.

I am also grateful that I have people who support me. Being involved in the Lupus Connection Support Group provides opportunities for me to communicate with others who have been diagnosed with lupus. The members are very supportive. My sister, who also has been diagnosed with lupus, is constantly encouraging me. My husband, my sister, and my mother are my main sources of daily support.

Thanks for reading my story. God bless!

My Lupie Bio

by Sarah Spadoni, CVT

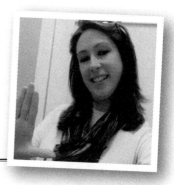

In 2007, I went to my regular doctor for a re-check on a urinary tract infection. I mentioned to her that I had been feeling exhausted and tired all the time, that I was having headaches a lot, and that I passed out on a regular basis. I was just going to chalk it up to being in school full-time and working part-time, but the doctor decided to do various tests to make sure everything looked okay.

"During the first of many visits, the rheumatologist completed an exam and more laboratory tests, but didn't find anything . . . so I went to a different medical facility. At the new offices, I saw more doctors who ordered more tests. They mentioned the word lupus, but never diagnosed me. "

My test results revealed that my health was kind of a mess. Some of my liver values were elevated. After completing more tests, the doctor determined that my liver was normal. However, she discovered that my heart had a small leak, but felt the leak was not enough to cause me to pass out. She also discovered that my antinuclear antibody was positive. That result signaled the possibility of my having an autoimmune disease, so the doctor referred me to a rheumatologist. That was the beginning of my four-year battle of trying to figure out what was wrong with me.

During the first of many visits, the rheumatologist completed an exam and more laboratory tests, but didn't find anything. She sent me home with a week of prednisone to see if that would help my headaches. Unfortunately, that did not help at all. I was not pleased with that doctor. I decided that I should see a more experienced rheumatologist, so I went to a differ- ent medical facility. At the new offices, I saw more doctors who ordered more tests. They mentioned the word lupus, but never diagnosed me. I took a break from these doctors and went on with my life, thinking that I might have this disease called lupus, but not knowing for sure.

I found a new doctor in 2008 and really trusted him. Well, my symptoms gradually got worse. I started a new job in October 2009. While I was employed there, I passed out on two occa- sions, and each time I was dizzy and nauseated for the rest of the day. I ended up going to the emergency room to try and get some relief. The ER doctors were able to treat the dizziness, but they provided no answers. I told them that I might have some autoimmune disease, but that didn't matter to them. I went home with a heart monitor, and that was all.

After getting rechecked every three months for a little over a year, I was finally given the diagnosis of systemic lupus erythe- matosus in 2011, a few days before my twenty-fourth birthday. I was actually happy to hear the diagnosis because it was such a huge relief knowing I wasn't losing my mind. I decided not to start any medication and just deal with the symptoms.

About six to ten months later my doctor convinced me to start Plaquenil, the go-to drug for lupus. Plaquenil is supposed to keep lupus from getting worse, and it has actually really helped my pain levels.

During all of this, my platelets were on a roller coaster ride and have gradually dropped all the way down to a concerning level. My understanding is that platelets help you clot and that if you don't have enough of them you have the risk of bleeding out. As of right now, the doctors are continuing to monitor them.

Lupus can cause so many different issues. It is a disease of so many faces. I feel it is going to get worse, but I refuse to let it claim who I am. I will fight it until the end!

Challenges to Remission; Hope for Removal

by Ivy M. Douglas

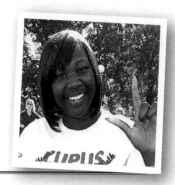

I was diagnosed with systemic lupus erythematosus in 2004 at the age of twenty-six. At that time, I was away at college preparing to graduate in less than two months with my master's degree in education.

For months, I had been experiencing extreme fatigue, and that had caused me a lot of problems with my student teaching. I would fall asleep every chance I got, whether I was in the classroom with the children or on my way to my classroom.

I had also been experiencing pain and swelling so bad that it was very difficult for me to get out of bed each morning. I would roll out of the bed to the floor and crawl to the bathroom. I would struggle to bend down to use the toilet. Painful and swollen hands presented another challenge as I tried to get dressed, especially with the buttons and zippers. It would take hours to get dressed, and I didn't have much help. I struggled trying to open and close doors. I really had a hard time trying to drive and get around. It would take a lot to start my car because I had problems turning the ignition key. Many times, I sat in my car, crying and praying trying to get the key to turn.

Once I accomplished that, I would make it to school and try to complete my student teaching for the day. It was a struggle

"Once I was diagnosed with lupus nephritis, my life began to change . . . I went from two prescriptions to more than ten pills a day. The doctors presented me with three different treatment plans for my diagnosis. Each plan was risky and had its own challenges. I was looking for the plan that would best fit my goal of being able to have children some day."

because my lesson plans required that I sit on the floor with my preschool children. Getting up and down was a major challenge and caused a decrease in my ability to perform at my best. My professors were not pleased with my performance. Therefore, the lupus caused me to have to repeat my class and extend my college career an additional semester.

There were several other symptoms I experienced as a result of lupus. Hair loss and weight fluctuation greatly influenced how I viewed myself. I have been wearing weaves and wigs ever since 2004. Due to the weight loss from the lupus and the weight gain from the prednisone, I have a closet with three different sizes of clothes.

After graduation, I worked in the child care field for seven years. Then my health issues worsened. In 2010, my kidneys began to be affected by the lupus, and I was diagnosed with lupus nephritis. I had several kidney biopsies that were painful and put me on bed rest for weeks. After getting results from the biopsies, I was informed that I was in stage three kidney disease and that my kidneys were functioning at only 23%. I was devastated and at a loss for words. I had been through several other biopsies on my neck, hand, and thyroid previously, but I had never received such negative results. And it was all due to lupus.

Once I was diagnosed with lupus nephritis, my life began to change. It started with my medications. I went from two prescriptions to more than ten pills a day. The doctors presented me with three different treatment plans for my diagnosis. Each plan was risky and had its own challenges. I was looking for the plan that would best fit my goal of being able to have children some day. Once I chose my plan, I was told that after the two-year process, my kidneys would be functioning at 60% or more. I was looking forward to achieving a higher level of kidney function, but I didn't realize what I was about to experience before I got there.

The first challenge I was to face was shingles. From my understanding, shingles is something that the elderly might experience, not a thirty-year-old. However, the Centers for Disease Control describes it as a painful skin rash caused by the same virus that causes chicken pox. I guess anyone can get it.

After that, I was in and out of the hospital because of low white and red blood cell counts. Then I had pneumonia. All this time, I was still trying to work as a preschool teacher. My body was in constant turmoil. I was fighting the germs from the preschoolers, fighting the stress of the job, and trying to adjust to the high doses of steroids.

During this time, my job did grant me short-term disability, but once it ended, I was in trouble again. I began to experience daily

> **"The first challenge I was to face was shingles . . . After that, I was in and out of the hospital because of low white and red blood cell counts. Then I had pneumonia. All this time, I was still trying to work as a preschool teacher. My body was in constant turmoil. I was fighting the germs from the preschoolers, fighting the stress of the job, and trying to adjust to the high doses of steroids . . . Then I was back to fighting low self-esteem again because of my appearance."**

lupus flares from head to feet, from swollen eyes to a balloon face. Then I was back to fighting low self-esteem again because of my appearance. I began to draw back from my regular activities and became confined to my house. I went from being a social butterfly to almost a hermit. Not only was my social life hindered, but my work life was also changing. I was unable to go to work and function for a full day due to the pain in my body and the extreme fatigue. Eventually, the doctors recommended that I resign from my job after being in the hospital over a week. It was really hard for me to resign because teaching was my passion, and I had worked so hard to earn my teaching certification. On top of that, I had been working since I was sixteen, so I couldn't imagine what I was going to do if I wasn't working.

Outside of working, I was also involved in my church. I was the youth pastor of my church for three years. When I stopped working, I also stepped back from ministry. Being the youth pastor was also a full-time job, but it was another passion of mine, and I enjoyed it. However, the stress and the time I needed to put in it were challenging due to the lupus. So, between not working and giving up ministry, I didn't have much of my life as I once knew it. Dealing with doctor appointments, medication, side effects from meds, and new symptoms consumed my day.

For months, the doctors made adjustments to my treatment plan in order to reduce the side effects of the meds. One of the side effects I experienced was insomnia, so I began seeing a doctor who specialized in sleep disorders. According to the sleep specialist, I was dealing with depression, and that condition played a major role in my sleep issue. As I sit here today and reflect on the things I have dealt with during this lupus journey, I can definitely say that I was depressed and at a point of giving up the fight.

After leaving my job, I then had to apply for disability. That was a challenge in itself, but I needed financial support, especially since I didn't have any insurance. My medical bills were piling up, and I also needed to pay for the many prescriptions I had to fill. The disability fight was a two-year battle. The disability doctor's argument was that because my kidney disease was not severe enough to warrant dialysis, I did not need disability. He stated that I could still work, just not in my field. I was very upset about that because I worked very hard to earn a degree and felt that my hard work earned me the right to work in my chosen field. So I started a legal battle to win disability benefits. After two years, I was finally approved. This was a huge stress relief. I was now able to focus on my health and not worry about paying for medical bills and medications.

I was recently informed that I am in remission, and I have been feeling a little better now. The main challenges I face today involve the many side effects of the medicines I am taking. I have started changing my eating habits. Plus, I have been exercising several days in the week. My biggest challenge right now is getting my kidneys functioning at a higher level so that I can stay away from dialysis. So, I am trusting in God and have faith that He will keep my lupus in remission until one day we find a cure.

The Bullet That Hit the Lupus Target

Unraveling the Mystery of the Role Lithium May Play in Creating Conditions for Developing Lupus

by Collette Clark

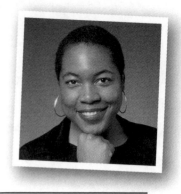

In the summer of my fourteenth year, a black cloud descends upon me. This dark specter wraps itself around me like a heavy dark cloak, dulling my emotions, stiffening my limbs, nearly extinguishing my spirit. That summer, sunlight causes physical pain and sears my eyes. I tack blankets to the windows to vanquish the enemy, making my room a still, dark tomb. I crawl into bed, burying myself under mounds of blankets, and sleep the whole summer away. These are the first signs of an old family curse, a curse that rears its head and possesses many of my relatives. These are the first signs of a bipolar disorder, then called manic depression.

Bipolar disorder is a mental illness that causes someone to experience extreme highs and lows. My mother is well acquainted with this old family foe. She recognizes the symptoms in me and immediately contacts her doctor for my treatment. The doctor experiments with a series of mood altering-drugs. Finally, we find a drug that seems to be the right stabilizing medication, "my savior," lithium.

Lithium succeeds at leveling my highs and lows, but my new companion seems to cause strange side effects. Pounds are poured onto my body, and my abdomen becomes swollen and distended. Each menstrual cycle is more painful and torturous than the last. It feels as though my legs don't belong to me and cause me to trip and slam into things. I feel nature's call, race to the bathroom, and nothing happens. I make endless hospital appointments about my health concerns, only to be to be told repeatedly:

"Miss Clark, there doesn't seem to be a problem."

"Miss Clark, everything seems okay."

"Miss Clark, we all have issues as we get older."

Then one year I experience a whole new set of strange symptoms. In the beginning of that year, I gain an enormous amount of weight. Almost overnight I become 218 pounds. I have a strange swollen appearance. My hands resemble hams. I lie in bed, feeling as if a semi-truck is on top of me. Only I am the truck! I become even more clumsy than usual. One day, I stand at the top of eight basement steps and fall straight down!

A sour taste of iron often invades my mouth. At times, I see things through a dim amber haze. Other times, I look around at nothing in particular, then suddenly, as if possessed, my eyes lock onto something and stare and stare and stare, like a hawk spotting prey. My mother suggests I hang some portraits I painted in my apartment. I am afraid to hang them; I don't like the way the people in the paintings stare at me. One night in the basement, I spot a fossilized mouse carcass embedded in the ceiling beams. I begin throwing newspapers at the mummified mouse, trying to dislodge it from the ceiling. Then I realize many hours later, that it is actually a wad of debris and spider webs.

"I make endless hospital appointments about my health concerns, only to be to be told repeatedly:

'Miss Clark, there doesn't seem to be a problem.'

'Miss Clark, everything seems okay.'

'Miss Clark, we all have issues as we get older.'"

Near the end of that year there is a drastic change in my weight. Pounds begin falling off me. Concerned, I make several hospital appointments. Each hospital weigh-in confirms numerous pounds melting at a rapid pace. I lose eighty-five pounds in three months!

Then one night I am startled awake from a deep sleep. I shoot straight up in bed, like I've been shocked by lightning. My brain sloshes around inside my skull like the liquid in a lava lamp. I fumble out of bed, moving like I'm trudging through waist high mud. My fingers are wet noodles as I finally hook my bra on the fifteenth try. I stumble on legs that move like a newborn calf. I shuffle downstairs, frantically shaking my bleary-eyed mom. Our car flies to the hospital.

After I am admitted to the hospital, the nurses draw blood and run some tests. Then, I am put into a room until someone is available to further assess me. I sit alone in the room viewing everything through a thick amber haze, my head bobbing up and down like a boat on troubled waters. Suddenly, a grim-faced doctor enters the room and says: "Miss Clark, you are experiencing a lithium toxicity."

My kidney function is down to forty percent. My kidneys are so damaged that the doctors think I will have to go on dialysis. Later on, an attendant enters the room to have me sign a consent form for an operation to remove the lithium from my body. After several tries, I can't get past the first three letters of my name! My brain is so fouled up I can't even remember how to spell my own name! I am admitted to the intensive care unit.

The ICU is shrouded in darkness, and the air is saturated with apprehension and doom, while I fight for my life. As my mom hovers over my bedside like a satellite, the hospital staff begins the process of removing my lithium, which triggers full-blown hallucinations. (The staring portraits and the mummified mouse were just the beginnings of them.) Over several days, my lithium-soaked mind waltzes between fantasy and reality. Each of the surreal episodes alternates with stretches of lucidity, only to be overtaken by the visions again. My hallucinations rival any sci-fi movie.

When I'm finally released to my mother and brought home, confusion still rules my mind. I flit between reality and fantasy. Am I really at home, or am I still at the hospital? My thirty-plus-year-old self sleeps next to my mother like a newborn.

Weeks after my toxicity episode, my mind and body betray me. A thick fog clouds my brain. My thoughts evaporate; words form, but come out as stutters. I can't read. I can't write. I can't draw. My sense of taste is warped. Sweet things are sourly bitter. All foods become unappetizing. If I am coaxed to eat anything, I can't keep it down. My rib bones protrude from my body.

Months after my toxicity episode, my sense of taste returns to normal, but I feel like a weed that has been broken down by wind and rain and is barely alive. To me, colors don't exist—just shades of grey. My bedroom is a cocoon where I sleep the day away. When I'm awake, my body violently rocks with tremors. Though my brain still refuses to hold a thought, at least the visions are gone. I am free from a long-term, ultimately abusive, relationship—I stop taking lithium.

More time passes. Once again my world has colors. My pencil writes stories. My pastels draw pictures. My mind comprehends and enjoys words. I seem to be returning to normal, but my intuition tells me I am forever changed. I'm still not in control. An unseen puppeteer holds the strings. This unseen force infuses searing pain into my joints, turning me into stone. We meet with my primary doctor about my symptoms. She suggests we see a specialist, a doctor who treats arthritis and other rheumatic conditions—a rheumatologist.

When we meet with the rheumatologist, he orders lab tests. When we see him again, the doctor gives the unseen puppeteer a name:

"Miss Clark, you have lupus. It is systemic."

The following years plunge me into a bad dream. It is a nightmare that ravages my body and batters my spirit. Lupus is a thug! It is a bully that plays with my body, like a deranged child plays with a new toy. The thieving wolf gnaws blinding pain into my legs (signs of kidney damage), stealing my sleep.

The puppeteer bows me over the toilet, making me heave and heave until my burning throat is raw and my churning stomach is empty. The unseen force stiffens my legs, making me use a walker. The thug paralyzes my legs with crippling arthritis, putting me in the hospital. The bully massacres many of my white blood cells, dangerously dwindling their numbers, once again depositing me in the hospital. Each hospital stay requires two blood transfusions. Lupus inflicts pain, bringing me to my knees, literally. I crawl like a baby up the three sets of stairs to my apartment. The wolf silences my left ear. Lupus carves disfiguring scars on my arms, pounds knots into my knuckles, twists my fingers into sickles, and forces me to wear the mask of the wolf.

Slowly, but surely, I begin to awaken from the bad dream. Just like when a stunted plant is deprived of sunlight and suddenly receives it, I slowly lift my head towards the light and begin to grow. It's now years since I've been a guest in a hospital room. At night, I am re-acquainted with my old friend, sleep. Sounds once again serenade my left ear. Even though I know he's still lurking, the wolf does not appear on my face. The arthritis that once rammed shards of pain into my joints, stiffening me into a statue, becomes a bad memory. Yet, I'm still submerged in sadness.

I realize I must fight this depression, and I start with my body. I exercise. Every single day, I fight. I shove back the covers. I punch down the gas pedal. I shuffle into the health club for my aerobic step class. At first my body is heavy and laden as I trip over my aerobic step. I move like a big ole' drowsy bear that just woke from a long hibernation. But, a year later, warmth and strength start swirling inside my body, spilling down my limbs to my fingertips and toes. My sneakers grow wings as I fly over my step.

I also improve my body by working on what I put in it, starting with one of my biggest indulgences—salt. In the good old days, I'd shake salt on each and every bite. Now, I peruse labels for low sodium, no salt added, and unsalted. Breakfast consists of hot, cooked cereals—oatmeal, barley, millet, and grits. Lunch includes leafy green salads, embellished with colorful vegetables, and drizzled with olive oil. Beef and milk rarely make an appearance. Adding kidney friendly foods to a diet already brimming with fruits and vegetables benefits my physical health. Cranberry juice is consumed three times a day. I make a conscious effort to drink water. And, when I do eat the bad stuff I plan for it every once in a while, not absent-mindedly all the time as I did in the past. The doctors add mycophenolate (CellCept) and lisinopril to my medicine regimen.

Another way to better health for me is to work on my emotional self. My attitude profoundly affects how my body copes with my illness. I know experiencing comradeship with others in the same trenches can only positively affect my disposition. I search for my people. I find them at Trinity.

The members of the Lupus Support Group at Trinity United Church of Christ welcome me with open arms. Looking into the faces of others who share my experiences comforts me. Hearing my stories echoing from the mouths of others is validating. At Trinity, I find encouragement, respect, and support. I am not alone. I feel my spirit rise.

I realize I have gifts to offer. I embrace my creativity by pursuing my three gifts: art, performing, and writing. I honor my art by joining Union Street Art Gallery, an environment that nurtures, honors, and shares creativity. I honor my performing by joining Toastmasters, a speaking group, where I learn how to effectively convey a message through the spoken word. My writing honors both my art and performing. Words are woven together forming speeches for performances. Words also become stories soon to be illustrated.

Now, my future appears on the horizon. It is bright, gleaming with possibilities, and radiating hope, like a sunrise signaling the start of a new day. As I become the author of my own story, by taking charge of my health and embracing my creativity, I start a new journey, pursuing the cause of my lithium toxicity—trying to unravel the mystery of the possible relationship between my lithium toxicity and my lupus. My concern with psychotropic drugs is not the drugs themselves. My issue is with how the drugs are being used. I believe that many of these drugs are not being properly monitored.

This is where I stand: I was diagnosed with lithium toxicity. Since I took lithium for twenty-two years (long-term), my toxicity would be defined as chronic, and I believe that the chronic lithium toxicity caused my lupus. Now, experts claim that if lupus is created due to a drug (in my case, maybe lithium), the damage done to the body reverses in a few weeks or months. This drug was pounding away at my kidney, thyroid, liver—my whole body—for over two decades. I propose that twenty-two years of damage is not going to reverse itself in a few weeks or months.

I have a theory as to how I developed lupus. The kidney and liver are the body's filtering organs. The thyroid affects the body's metabolism. If not properly monitored, lithium can cause damage to these organs. Damage to these systems affects how the body fights toxins, viruses, germs, etc. and how the body's other organs and systems do their jobs. The damage can appear in the body in many ways. I believe my damage expresses itself through my immune system as lupus.

By telling my story, I hope to participate in the dialogue about the proper monitoring of psychotropic drugs. I want my experience to be one of the catalysts making lithium toxicities—which may contribute to development of lupus—a thing of the past. Because of my experience with lithium and lupus, I urge those taking psychotropics (and other drugs) to analyze and save all test results. We should develop a partnership with our doctors so that we can diligently monitor how the drugs are affecting our organs and general health.

I believe that my time on lithium, my lithium toxicity, and my lupus are woven together tightly like a tapestry. I believe it is a tapestry that is woven for thousands each year. This must stop! If it turns out that a drug causing damage to the kidney, liver, and thyroid has no connection to an autoimmune disease like lupus, which also may cause damage to the kidney, liver, and thyroid, then I feel that my lithium toxicity definitely didn't help! I believe, with every fiber of my being, that my lithium toxicity is the Bullet That Hit the Lupus Target. My intuition tells me so!

Resilient

by Sherron N. Buford

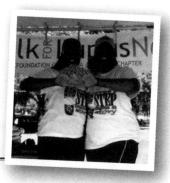

How could a twenty-six-year-old young woman who didn't smoke, who never took any type of birth control, and who never had surgery or any major medical issues develop quarter-sized blood clots in her lungs? After my two-week stay in the hospital, the doctors concluded that the reason was lupus. That was in April 2008. I will never forget the day, time, or location when my life changed forever.

Around January 2008, after losing up to forty pounds by exercising and eating right, I started to feel extremely tired for no apparent reason. I noticed that my left hand would turn blue and would be almost numb to the touch for days at a time. A small red butterfly-shaped rash surfaced across the bridge of my nose. I thought it was due to exercising. I would cough uncontrollably, trying to catch my breath after walking only a short distance. I asked myself, "Why am I feeling so bad when this is the best shape I've been in for more than four or five years?" I knew something was wrong and that I had to have it checked out immediately because I was never sick.

I visited the doctor five times in a three-month time span when I first realized something was wrong. During those three months, I was diagnosed as having everything from an upper respiratory infection, to bronchitis, to pneumonia. However, more tests and scans were done that determined I had pulmonary embolisms (blood clots in my lungs). I was frustrated and angry because I wanted answers to the many questions going through my mind. Why wasn't I tested for it? Why did it take my going to the doctors five times before being diagnosed? What if I hadn't been persistent in going back to the doctors when I knew something wasn't right? TO GOD BE THE GLORY!

It is suspected that people inherit something from their parents that predisposes them to develop lupus. They are not necessarily pre-destined to develop lupus, but they may be more susceptible.

Although it has never been discovered that anyone in my family was diagnosed with lupus, the above statistic is of high concern for me because I have an identical twin sister who could most likely be at risk of developing lupus as well. Because she shows very few signs or symptoms, doctors are unable to diagnose her as having lupus. Doctors can only treat patients once they show enough symptoms to be diagnosed. There isn't any kind of preventive treatment that she can take. It's a wait-and-see

In studies of identical twins, when one twin has lupus, the other twin has a 24-percent chance of developing it. This and other research suggests that genetics plays an important role, but it also shows that genes alone do not determine who gets lupus, and that other factors play a role.[30]

type of approach where we can only monitor to see if she'll show more symptoms. All of our lives, my sister and I have often had to share just about everything. But lupus is one thing I wouldn't mind keeping to myself.

After leaving the hospital, the journey of learning how to cope and adjust to life with lupus began. It was alarming and surreal for me to hear that at the age of twenty-six I would be on medications such as warfarin and Plaquenil for the rest of my life. The combination of these medications wreaked havoc on my skin, hair, and digestive system. It took me quite some time to find the balance of how to function in the world while dealing with lupus flares. Although I have a twin sister with whom I've been blessed to share my life's deepest thoughts, pains, and pleasures, I couldn't begin to describe what I was going through as I started to cope with lupus. Lupus is an isolating disease, and it left me feeling (and at times I still feel) ALONE.

My faith in God is what sustains me in my everyday walk of life. My relationship with God continues to give me the strength, courage, and confidence to wake up each day with a positive outlook about my circumstances and about everything (good or bad) that has taken place in my life. I realize that at one point in my life, I almost didn't wake up. So I'm grateful for each breath that God allows me to take, for each breath serves a purpose.

After attending the funeral of a very close childhood friend who died in June 2011 from complications due to lupus, I feel that I have no choice but to live each day with purpose, not just for me but for her, my sister, friends, and millions of others who are affected or impacted by lupus. I rebuke the potential for lupus

"After leaving the hospital, the journey of learning how to cope and adjust to life with lupus began. It was alarming and surreal for me to hear that at the age of twenty-six I would be on medications such as warfarin and Plaquenil for the rest of my life. The combination of these medications wreaked havoc on my skin, hair, and digestive system. It took me quite some time to find the balance of how to function in the world while dealing with lupus flares."

to hinder my life in any way. By God's stripes, I am healed.

Today, I encourage others and actively participate in various lupus awareness initiatives. I volunteer for the Lupus Society of Illinois at area health fairs, and I participate in awareness walks. These are avenues I use in striving to spread the word and to encourage others to get in the loop about lupus.

Navigating the Path Toward Health and Wellness

by Richard Mebane

I consider my story a more fortunate one compared to many others. I was already on a path toward a health and wellness career when my lupus symptoms developed. I was always a pretty athletic and physically active person. At around thirty years old, I had gotten a little overweight and out of shape. So in 2000, I resolved to get back in shape, and in 2001, I became an avid runner and ran my first marathon. By 2004, I had run my seventh marathon. I had actually started developing symptoms while training for three back-to-back marathons but managed to tough it out.

While building up for my next marathon, my symptoms overwhelmed my body. Fatigue set in. I went from being able to run as many miles as I wanted to barely being able to run one mile. I was waking up with my arms completely numb and hands swollen. I had mysterious bruises on the top of my head. I would joke that my wife was beating me up in my sleep. I started to take the situation seriously when back spasms forced me to the emergency room. My primary physician at the time told me to stop exercising so much and that I was just getting older, even though I was only thirty-four years old. He diagnosed me with arthritis and prescribed ibuprofen and muscle relaxers. I was still getting the back spasms that made breathing difficult. The muscle relaxers made me feel like a zombie, so I tried physical therapy, which helped some.

"I was already on a path toward a health and wellness career when my lupus symptoms developed. I went from being able to run as many miles as I wanted to barely being able to run one mile. I was waking up with my arms completely numb and hands swollen. I had mysterious bruises on the top of my head. I would joke that my wife was beating me up in my sleep. I started to take the situation seriously when back spasms forced me to the emergency room."

Finally, my wife convinced me to see a different doctor she heard about from one of her coworkers who had a similar experience. Through the grace of God, this new doctor knew just enough about lupus to refer me to a rheumatologist. The rheumatologist ran a series of tests and within a couple of visits was able to confirm my condition as systemic lupus erythematosus in November 2005. For me, the lupus diagnosis was a great relief. I felt that once I knew what was wrong, I could figure out what to do next. It was extremely frustrating dealing with doctors who didn't have a clue as to what was happening to my body. When my rheumatologist explained to me what lupus is, I had just recently become a full-time personal trainer. Therefore, I felt I was in a good position to make the right lifestyle changes that I would need to fight back. I was also encouraged by the fact that my new rheumatologist was also a marathon runner and understood my psychological need to be physically active. He also pointed out that we caught this in its early stages, which meant I stand a great chance of living a normal and productive life. I may even be able to run another marathon some day.

What I didn't anticipate was how my family would react. My wife, my parents, and siblings were very upset and concerned. When I broke the news to my wife (over the phone), I was so excited to finally get an understanding of what was going on with my health, that I didn't realize how worried she was until she showed up less than an hour later in tears. My mother and sister had similar reactions. Eventually, I was able to reassure everyone that I would be all right and that I was very fortunate to get diagnosed so early while still in relatively good health.

My lupus diagnosis created some very positive changes in my life. One, it changed how I manage my healthcare. I consider myself to be an athletic person and will only take advice from medical professionals who are athletic or trained to advise athletes. Two, I take my health much more seriously and now realize that I am not invincible. Three, I changed my professional focus to helping others improve their health. I've been a certified fitness instructor for almost ten years now. For the last three years, I have been focusing on helping chiropractic patients heal and improve the quality of their lives. I am currently in school to become a licensed occupational therapy assistant and eventually, a physical therapist. I hope to increase my opportunities to help others to live and enjoy healthier and more fruitful lives.

Like I stated in the beginning, I realize that I am extremely fortunate and blessed. Hopefully my story can give strength to help someone less fortunate.

My Life With Lupus
(Blessed; Not Broken)

by Kanefus R. Walker

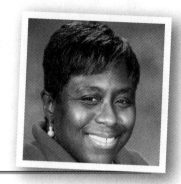

My recollection of the initial stages of lupus began at the beginning of 2009. My symptoms began with usual fatigue here and there. Then I started noticing my hands swelling and stiffening to the point where my knuckles were turning black. My bedroom at home was on the second floor, so daily I made trips up and down the stairs for whatever I needed, be it going to the refrigerator, going out the door, or participating in simple family time. My time upstairs usually consisted of enjoying my alone time, going to bed for the night, or hanging-out time when I had company over.

On New Year's Eve 2008, my brother proposed to his now-wife with our family present. Once she said yes, we knew the next thing on the agenda would be wedding plans. My now-sister-in-law asked me to be a bridesmaid in their wedding. I have a history of being overweight, so I had to do something about that to look good for my brother's June nuptials. In February 2009, I began my weight loss journey. At the time, I was out of work, so my workout regimen was very rigid. I began working out every day, sometimes twice a day. I watched very closely what I ate, making sure that I did what was necessary to peel those pounds off. As the weight began to come off, I could see the results beginning to form, and it only made me work out all the more.

Around April 2009, I began to notice that going up and down the stairs had become a slight challenge and that being tired became an issue. Each day, activities that usually took very little time began to take more time. But I ignored it because I was looking good as my weight loss was really taking shape. When I went places, I would get looks and sometimes even second looks and a lot of compliments, especially from people who knew my struggle.

Fast forward to June 2009. I was a bridesmaid in my brother's wedding, and many spoke about how good I looked after my weight loss. However, something just wasn't right. My hands had begun to swell slowly, my knees ached, and walking was feeling a little different. But hey, I ignored it and kept going. Nothing was keeping me down. I was on a mission, and so far, this time I had been more successful than in all my previous attempts at losing weight.

At that time, I was a thirty-nine-year-old, single female living at home with my parents. Because I lived at home, my mother, who is my real doctor, was able to notice some changes in me. She asked me about the changes, and I described what I was going through. I was reminded that I come from a family of lupus patients. I have a sister, three brothers and a niece who have all been diagnosed and living daily with this disease. My mother stated that my symptoms mirrored those of my sister's prior to her lupus diagnosis. Therefore, she believed that I had lupus also. Of course, we were not 100% sure that I had lupus; it was a mama's hunch.

I struggled as my condition got worse. Every day, going up and

"I struggled as my condition got worse. Every day, going up and down the stairs had become an arduous task . . . When taking a bath, getting in the tub was easy; getting out was another story . . . Opening a simple bottle of water was impossible. My body began to stiffen all over to the point where walking was no longer easy. Needless to say, my workouts were no longer possible. That became depressing because I still didn't really know what the problem was."

down the stairs had become an arduous task. It became so bad that each day I had to develop ways of limiting the number of times I needed to navigate the stairs. One thing that helped a lot was to bring everything that I needed downstairs with me in the morning and stay down until bedtime. When taking a bath, getting in the tub was easy; getting out was another story. Since my hands were not strong enough to support my weight, I would use my forearms when getting out of the tub. Opening a simple bottle of water was impossible. My body began to stiffen all over to the point where walking was no longer easy. Needless to say, my workouts were no longer possible. That became depressing because I still didn't really know what the problem was.

I woke up one Thursday morning and decided I had experienced enough. I could barely turn my head, so I knew I needed to see someone. During this time, I was unemployed, so my only option was to go to the emergency room at Oak Forest Hospital, a division of Cook County Hospital System. When I finally saw an ER doctor, he looked at me and virtually said nothing was really wrong. He advised me to take some Tylenol, and stated that "it" would go away. What the hell is "it"?! I was not satisfied, but did not feel well enough to argue or question him, so I did the best I could at that time—I went home. Well, that proved futile because my symptoms only worsened, and I found myself back at the ER the next day, making sure I saw anybody except the doctor from the previous day.

Another ER doctor took one look at me, saw my swollen hands and stiff walk, and decided to run some tests. Finally, someone with half a brain showed some concern. He said that he thought I might have lupus, but because he was an ER physician, he was not permitted to make any type of diagnosis. Therefore, he ordered some blood work and a urinalysis. I was to come back to see him. Each trip to the ER got harder, to the point where a two-minute walk from my car took ten minutes. Finally, it took so much for me to walk and drive, I decided to try to reach him by telephone. After what seemed like a million phone calls, I decided the only thing I could do was go back to the ER and try to catch him.

I returned to the ER again only to find out that the doctor had gone on vacation out of the country and wouldn't be back for another week. What am I supposed to do now? Could I deal with this another week, waiting for some results? So I still had to return to the ER one more time.

Finally, I was able to see another ER doctor who was able to review my results. She looked at me, and like the previous doctor, said she also believed I had lupus but was unable to diagnose. She called Cook County Hospital herself and scheduled my appointment with a rheumatologist. There was a long waiting list of patients to see the rheumatologist, so I still had about another two weeks before I could see the doctor.

Finally, July 20 came, and I was able to see the rheumatologist. The diagnosis was systemic lupus erythematosus (SLE). Lupus was not new to me. My sister and my niece have SLE, and my three brothers have discoid lupus. So that day, I became the sixth member of my immediate family to receive a diagnosis of this disease. I have seen my sister and my niece struggle to the point of almost dying, then being able to bounce back into remission. Unlike them, I feel my case of lupus is a milder form. The worst part of dealing with this was the initial flare and not knowing what was really going on. The inability to walk unnerved me, but I took it in stride. All I could say was that my mama was right the whole time.

The first thing my rheumatologist did was put me on prednisone, Plaquenil, and a vitamin-D and calcium combination. The prednisone, of course is a steroid, so there went all of my hard work and dedication to eating right and exercising down the drain. Because I have been eating everything that isn't nailed down, I have gone back to struggling with my weight. I still try to work out when I can. Although I try to make healthy eating choices, I am not always successful. It is a daily work in progress.

I had the same rheumatologist from the beginning of my diagnosis until last year. Due to personal obligations, she had to relocate. I was sad that I had to make the change because I felt it left me vulnerable to someone that I wasn't sure would measure up to my standards. We are fighting a disease that is killing us from the inside out, and most don't seem to understand that except the people who are affected by it. As a person with lupus, you are not able to talk to everyone about your disease. I know that I'm dealing with a horrible disease that is very unpredictable, so building trust and establishing a partnership with my medical provider are two very important issues for me. When I found a doctor who I felt was passionate enough about this disease and my well-being and care, it was very important to have her in my life and on my care team. Luckily, my new rheumatologist is just as committed to this disease as my former one. So I am happy with her.

At first, I was interested in increasing lupus awareness because some of my family members had been diagnosed. Then, receiving my own diagnosis made me push all the more. I started attending a lupus support group. Currently, I am the group leader of The Lupus Connection, sponsored by the Lupus Society of Illinois (LSI). I am inspired when I hear others share their stories. I see that they are going through so much more than I am. I can't help but be grateful of where I am with this disease.

I became extremely active with the lupus walk in my area. I even serve as co-captain of my own walk team, **Flare Fighters**. I have also hosted health fairs and invited representatives from LSI to share information about lupus. Involvement of this kind prompted a group of us to organize an annual holiday fundraiser, Holiday Dreams—Cure for Lupus Dinner Dance. I feel I have to get the word out by any means necessary.

For about four years, I was flare-free. However, over the last three months, I have been bothered with rashes off and on. That's an indication that my lupus has become active again. I still take Plaquenil and the vitamin-D/calcium combination. Now, I am also taking methotrexate and folic acid to help with the rash. I am not happy to have to add to my medicine cocktail, but I have to do what is necessary to continue in this fight.

My faith in God helps me so much. My active lifestyle with the church keeps me balanced so that depression and all of the other negatives do not set in. God is truly my source of strength. Reading my Bible daily gives me the comfort that I need.

Lupus is not a death sentence for everyone. Although many struggle, many others go on to live full lives, have children, raise families, have careers, etc. I salute those who have passed on, and I embrace those who are newly diagnosed. I urge education for those who know nothing of the disease or how to help those with it. I fight for awareness and hope that lupus becomes as important as cancer, heart disease, and all of the other more commonly-known health challenges. I walk with and for those of us who, on the outside, "don't look sick" but on the inside are being torn apart. My life with lupus is still being lived. I have been blessed to be able to go and do as I did before my diagnosis.

Lupus has not broken me.

Part 4
Stories About Lupus Warriors Diagnosed Later In Life

In the pamphlet *Many Shades*, the NIH reports that many people have lupus for a long time before they receive an accurate diagnosis. One reason may be that there is no single test that can determine whether a person has lupus.[31] Usually, doctors will do a complete physical exam, run several laboratory tests of blood and urine samples, study the medical history, and may also do a biopsy of skin or kidney tissue. It may take time for the doctor to gather all the information, analyze the results, rule out other possible diagnoses, and determine that one definitely has lupus.[32] In the meantime, lupus symptoms may come and go over time.[33]

According to the American College of Rheumatology, if the physician finds that a patient is experiencing at least four of the symptoms listed below, and finds no other reason for them, the patient may be diagnosed with lupus:[34]

Rashes:
- butterfly-shaped rash over the cheeks—referred to as malar rash
- red rash with raised round or oval patches—known as discoid rash
- rash on skin exposed to the sun

Mouth sores: sores in the mouth or nose lasting from a few days to more than a month

Arthritis: tenderness and swelling lasting for a few weeks in two or more joints

Lung or heart inflammation: swelling of the tissue lining the lungs (referred to as pleurisy or pleuritis) or the heart (pericarditis), which can cause chest pain when breathing deeply

Kidney problem: blood or protein in the urine, or tests that suggest poor kidney function

Neurologic problems: seizures, strokes or psychosis (a mental health problem)

Abnormal blood tests:
- low blood cell counts: anemia, low white blood cells or low platelets
- positive antinuclear antibody: referred to as ANA and present in nearly all patients with lupus
- certain antibodies that show an immune system problem: anti-double-strand DNA (called anti-dsDNA), anti-Smith (referred to as anti-Sm) or antiphospholipid antibodies, or a false-positive blood test for syphilis (meaning you do not really have this infection)

NIH points out that because the symptoms vary with individuals and could be mistaken for other diseases, patients could "go for months or years without an accurate diagnosis."[35]

The Latest Leg of My Journey

by Jameela Lindsey

Being diagnosed with systemic lupus erythematosus in 1999 has really been a challenge for me. Over the years, there have been many symptoms and continued usage of various medications for relief. It takes time to find out what combination of medicines will work best. It took a couple of years for me.

I have learned to expect the unexpected, and I ask myself all the time, "What will I go through next?" God has been by my side, taking me through it all, whether it's joint pain, kidney failure, or just plain being tired. I am writing today about the most recent leg of my journey.

In May 2012, my husband and I took a trip to Maryland to visit relatives. We arrived safely and were having a wonderful visit. One night, we went to the movies, and I enjoyed some popcorn and pop. This was nothing unusual. The next morning I woke up with intense stomach pains and made a trip to the nearest urgent care clinic.

The doctor gave me some medicine to ease the pain temporarily. After the drive back to Illinois, I had my husband drive me straight to the emergency room. It turns out that I had diverticulitis (inflammation of the intestine) with an abscess in my colon. With continual stomach pains, I ended up in the hospital for a week and a half while the doctors tried to dissolve the abscess with antibiotics. When that didn't work, surgery was the next step.

Could lupus be attacking my colon? The doctors never said it was, so I really don't know. But with lupus, anything can happen.

On September 19, 2012, the abscess was removed, but I had to wear a colostomy bag. According to Medline Plus from the Internet, "Colostomy is a surgical procedure that brings one end of the large intestine out through an opening (stoma) made in the abdominal wall. Stools moving through the intestine drain through the stoma into a bag attached to the abdomen."[36]

What a new experience for me! Trial and error kicked in. Leaks brought embarrassment and frustration. But by the grace of God, I was able to find the right fit that was comfortable to me. As time passed, I was able to get into a normal routine of maintaining the bag.

Normally, a second surgery is done in about five or six months to reverse the colostomy and reattach the colon, but I was not ready physically or emotionally. I had to ask myself, "Is my body ready for another surgery? Will the lupus start to flare?"

Family members wanted me to have the surgery done right away. Despite what anyone said, I had to be the one to decide. Prayers to God helped me to make that decision. On October 1, 2013, I had my second surgery. It's now been four months since the surgery, and I am still healing. With the support of The Lupus Connection (my support group) and family members, I am able to continue on a day-to-day basis. I handle each day as it

"I have learned to expect the unexpected, and I ask myself all the time, 'What will I go through next?' God has been by my side, taking me through it all, whether it's joint pain, kidney failure, or just plain being tired."

comes, and I thank God for enabling me to manage. I have faith that His grace and mercy will see me through any new episode that awaits me on my journey. I look to and depend on Him. He is my rock and never leaves me.

Armed With Hope and Knowledge

by Tari Ambler

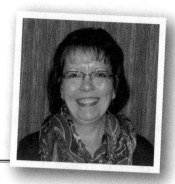

Ihave been living with systemic lupus erythematosus since November 1996. I guess I was lucky in that it only took about eight months for me to get the diagnosis of lupus nephritis as an answer to the problems I was having. Some of my symptoms were: costochondritis (inflammation of the chest wall), joint pain, swollen lymph nodes, and Raynaud's Syndrome (decrease in blood flow, usually to fingers and toes). I even had to endure a lymph node biopsy for lymphoma in the spring of 1996. Thankfully that came back benign, but it did show general inflammation, which the doctor ignored. I was so happy I didn't have lymphoma that I let the information about the inflammation slide.

Then in September 1996, I got really sick and was diagnosed with Epstein-Barr mono. According to Medline Plus, mono is usually linked to the Epstein-Barr virus.[37] The CDC says Epstein-Barr virus is one of the most common viruses to infect humans and can cause symptoms such as fatigue, fever, sore throat, swollen lymph nodes, and rash.[38]

As the weeks went by with no relief, a new doctor started to run all kind of tests. These test results ultimately led her to tentatively diagnose me with SLE. That call came on my thirty-eighth birthday, not exactly a present I was thrilled with! I was then sent to a nephrologist (a doctor who specializes in diseases of the kidney) because of my extreme proteinuria (excessive amount of protein in the urine). My kidneys were biopsied right before Thanksgiving, and my diagnosis was officially membranous lupus nephritis.

My worst flare came in the summer of 2000 and resulted in another kidney biopsy. Unfortunately, I had internal kidney bleeding as a side effect, then ended up in the hospital after taking naproxen for the severe kidney pain. My creatinine levels (an indication of poor kidney function) went dangerously high, and I developed fluid imbalance. I was very sick, even to the point where I was truly scared for my life.

Though my kidney function improved enough to be released from the hospital, my severe edema continued. I was unable to wear shoes because of my swollen feet, and I would wake up with such facial edema that one eye was swollen shut. The treatment from my local nephrologist gave me no relief. It was not until I switched to a new nephrologist at a teaching hospital that I started on the road to recovery.

I have learned that my kidneys can't tolerate any nonsteroidal anti-inflammatory drugs (NSAIDs), which are included in the treatment plan for many lupus patients. Soon after that hospitalization, I was started on Enalapril, an ACE inhibitor—a drug used to treat high blood pressure, congestive heart failure, swelling, and rheumatoid arthritis—to control inflammation in my kidneys. I also began tapering off of prednisone. The treatment plan was for me to start on another immune suppressant.

However, miraculously, my kidney function began to improve so that by the time my prednisone dose was zero, I didn't need to start on another immune suppressant. Luckily, I haven't experienced anything as serious as that again. I hope I never will.

Since then, my road has sometimes been filled with potholes but also many smooth patches. I was on prednisone for more than five years and suffer from osteopenia (decreased bone density) as a result. Prednisone can save your life, but the side effects can also make it miserable. I'm lucky that I never had to be on some of the more toxic chemotherapeutic drugs that may be used to treat lupus.

Even though I have coped with a chronic illness for more than seventeen years, I have to say my life is better because of it. One of the first thoughts I had when I was diagnosed was that I might not even see my children grow up. During those first scary weeks, our wonderful families and those at our church embraced our family with love, support, prayers and meals. After several months, I decided, with God's help, I was going to manage this illness and do what I could to live normally. I knew I would have to keep a positive attitude if I was going to be successful. We learned how to accept help from others. My husband, Dale, started to research SLE and learned that it is a chronic condition that can be managed. My mother-in-law always told me that God doesn't give us more than we can handle. I think sometimes He has more confidence in us than we have in ourselves. My fears began to turn into determination. My faith has grown stronger since then, and I try to help others whenever I can. I'm not sure how we could have managed

"My advice to lupus patients is, if possible, be under the care of a rheumatologist and other specialists as your individual case dictates. It is vitally important to find the right doctor and/or specialist for your case. So don't be afraid to switch to one with whom you can have a good relationship. Having sufficient health insurance coverage, one that allows the lupus patient to see specialists as needed, is very important as well."

without support from others, so I try to pass that help along.

I am so thankful to have been in remission since 2006, having very few symptoms and leading a healthy life. I have two adult children and have been married to my wonderfully supportive husband, Dale, for more than thirty-one years. My family and friends are more precious to me. Everyone has been so supportive of me and given me a reason to stay well.

I am thankful that my background in the healthcare field has helped me in coping with my illness. I did a lot of reading and research on nutrition in relation to disease. With the help of a nutritionist, I started on a path of following a healthy diet and taking supplements. When I was able, I resumed my physical activity. I believe in an integrated approach to dealing with my lupus. My approach includes using good medical specialists, balanced nutrition (including supplements), regular exercise, yoga, and chiropractic care.

My feeling is that most general practitioners aren't usually trained sufficiently to treat autoimmune diseases such as lupus. My advice to lupus patients is, if possible, be under the care of a rheumatologist and other specialists as your individual case dictates. It is vitally important to find the right doctor and/ or specialist for your case. So don't be afraid to switch to one with whom you can have a good relationship. Having sufficient health insurance coverage, one that allows the lupus patient to see specialists as needed, is very important as well.

Becoming knowledgeable about SLE helped me in so many ways in the early years after my diagnosis. I was able to learn about the various blood tests, diagnostic tests, and how to better nourish my body with good food. I became interested in more ways to help myself and others deal with lupus. I started attending a local lupus support group and took on the leadership of it in 2002. I became a support group leader to help the Lupus Society of Illinois to fulfill their purpose of providing resources for the lupus community.

I try to tell anyone who is newly diagnosed to please not ignore it. Take ownership and control of your illness, and with the help of health professionals, make the changes that give you improvement. I enjoy talking to lupus patients and their families, and I want to give them hope. Armed with hope and knowledge, we can live a better tomorrow.

Living Well With Lupus

by Kay Mimms

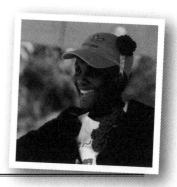

I awake in my own bed, open my eyes, and discover the need to use the bathroom. It's Monday, November 24, 2008, around 5:30 a.m., and as I do most mornings, I thank the Lord for allowing me to be able to use the bathroom without having to wait for someone to take me. This is about the same time I would wake up when I was a patient at the Rehabilitation Institute of Chicago (RIC). Back then, I was unable to walk, could barely talk, and had to be assisted with most jobs. I had a catheter, but I didn't want to be embarrassed by dirtying my diaper. So I would wait to hear the sound of the blood pressure cart being pushed down the hall. *Screeech! Screeeech! Screeeeech! Screeeeech! Screeeeeech!* I would say to myself, "How much longer before she reaches my room? Will I be able to hold it?"

I knew that even if I tried to call the nurses before the aide reached me, either they would ignore my call or would probably not be able to understand what I wanted. You see, I could only whisper, and most times people at the nurses' station would forget that fact and probably think that someone was just playing with the call button. I knew the aide would have to take my blood pressure and administer my first medication by 6:30 a.m. So I would just lie there, anxiously waiting and hoping that I could hold out until she arrived.

For years, probably my whole life, I suffered with various symptoms that could have been related to lupus. My symptoms included cold hands and feet and sensitivity to cold (since I can remember); painful, sore, and swollen joints and muscles (since the 1960s); low blood count (1960s); extreme redness of eyes (since 1975); thyroid condition (since 1988); itchy and discolored blotches on skin (1990s); blistering after short exposure to sun (1990s); chest pain with each deep breath (1990s); itchy, flaky scalp (2005); hair loss (2005); loss of appetite (2005); and extreme fatigue (2005).

All those years, my doctors did a good job of treating my symptoms; however, many times either the old symptoms would just reappear, or I'd get new ones. My dermatologists and ophthalmologist even recommended evaluations for lupus at different times. I followed their recommendations, but the results were always negative. I discovered later that I didn't have enough markers—the magic number being four simultaneous symptoms—to determine a definite lupus diagnosis. I just continued seeing doctors whenever conditions warranted such. Therefore, I was able to continue my career in education as the doctors tried to keep my symptoms under control. Then in 2004, I retired after more than thirty years of continuous, successful employment.

When I first retired, life was beautiful. I spent my days being involved in many activities that I was not able to do while working. I exercised four days a week, had breakfasts and lunches with my retired buddies, took advantage of free seminars and workshops, participated in two book clubs, and took at least one cruise or some other extended vacation once a year. I had it all planned out.

Then in 2005, the health issues that had aggravated me for decades exacerbated, and some new ones came along. I was losing hair. I had to force myself to eat because all food tasted like metal or just had no taste at all, so I was losing weight. This wasn't so bad as I had always wanted to lose some weight. However, I knew I needed nourishment in order to maintain some degree of my health, so I forced myself to eat, even if nothing but soups. I was tired all the time. I would drag myself to the gym, drag myself back home, and then just vegetate on the sofa for hours.

I discovered that things were really bad while we were on an extended cruise in the Caribbean, as I detailed earlier in the book. One night after dinner, I tried to stand so that we could return to our cabin. To my and everyone else's surprise, I could

---

"My symptoms included cold hands and feet and sensitivity to cold (since I can remember); painful, sore, and swollen joints and muscles (since the 1960s); low blood count (1960s); extreme redness of the eyes (since 1975); thyroid condition (since 1988); itchy and discolored blotches on skin (1990s); blistering after short exposure to sun (1990s); chest pain with each deep breath (1990s); {and since 2005} itchy, flaky scalp, hair loss, loss of appetite and extreme fatigue."

---

barely stand and had much difficulty walking. My husband, Cecil, had to help me walk to our cabin. I was also very cold and ached all over. I used aspirin to try to ward off the pain in my muscles and joints. Then, even though the temperature was in the 80s outside, we switched our thermostat from the air conditioner to the heat. I still was not able to get warm, so I put on more clothing and covered myself with extra blankets. Poor Cecil! I felt sorry for him. He loves the cool air, yet he had to suffer through the night in a hot cabin.

After that experience, I was determined to find out what was happening to me. When we got home, I pressed my doctors to do a more thorough investigation of my symptoms. That started a battery of tests, including a bone marrow biopsy. That was very painful, but I was glad about the negative results. Doctors researched many avenues, but failed to solve the mystery of my complaints. My condition was getting worse, so our cousin, Dr. Alfred Cook, recommended one of his colleagues who seems to love the challenge of solving medical puzzles and appears to go after medical mysteries with a vengeance. His name is Dr. Michael Zielinski; I call him Dr. Z.

Dr. Z gave me a thorough exam and asked many questions. His first conclusion was that I might have sarcoidosis, but he wanted to do more tests. Before we left his office that day, he looked into my eyes and said with emphasis, "We *are* going to find out what's wrong with you." I felt very confident that he would follow through with his promise.

On my way home, I thought, "Sarcoidosis. *What* is that?!" I started doing research, and I didn't like what I discovered. Sarcoidosis causes inflammation, most often seen in the lungs, lymph nodes, and skin. It starts as tiny lumps called granulomas,[39] the result of cells—sent out by the body's immune system in response to an unknown substance detected in the body—sticking together and forming a lump.[40] Symptoms can include cough, shortness of breath, weight loss, and fatigue.[41] But at least with a diagnosis of sarcoidosis I had a possible answer for my health concerns.

Dr. Z called me a few days later. My results showed that my thyroid was normal; however, my blood count was still low. He also said that sarcoidosis was less likely. Whew! I escaped that bullet. But what *is* the problem? He wanted me to do the anti-nuclear antibody test for systemic arthritis. This test confirmed that I have lupus. Finally, in February 2006, at the age of fifty-nine, I was given the proper diagnosis—LUPUS. That was hard to accept, especially since I had two nieces who had died after suffering complications from lupus. I was scared, yet I felt that now at least we knew what was wrong with me, and maybe I could get proper treatment and survive. Some time later, I remember hearing that in my case, I had to be in a flare in order for the doctors to make a definite lupus diagnosis. Am I special, or what?

Dr. Z referred me to Dr. Rosalind Ramsey-Goldman, who is a rheumatologist, an esteemed lupus researcher, and the chief investigator for Northwestern University's Patient-Oriented Clinical Research Program in Lupus. I took the first available appointment with her for Tuesday, February 14, two weeks after my lupus diagnosis. However, before my scheduled appointment, my condition worsened. I experienced nausea, more pain and swelling, difficulty in mobility, and deep coughs that produced pinkish mucous.

What a mess! I thought. I wanted to keep my appointment with Dr. Ramsey-Goldman, but I didn't think I could stand this pain any longer. Also, why was I coughing up this pink stuff? Did I have an ulcer?

These additional symptoms led me to the hospital emergency room where doctors discovered crackles in my lungs and an elevated troponin level, revealing possible damage to my heart. This made them suspect pericardial and pleural effusion (fluid around the heart and lungs). I was admitted to the hospital.

Later that night, I began coughing up blood and experienced acute respiratory distress, hypotension (low blood pressure), presumed seizure, and loss of consciousness. The medical staff ordered a respiratory code (breathing and possible airway blockage emergency), blood type and crossmatching, intubation, and sedation. Later, I think the conclusion was as follows: there was bleeding in my lungs, and the heparin (blood thinner) that was administered for possible heart problems caused my lungs to hemorrhage. In my heart of hearts, I feel that had I not been in the hospital, I would have died that very night. As my body slowly tried to heal, I remained in the intensive care unit, intubated and sedated off and on, for more than sixty days.

In April, I was finally weaned from the ventilator; however, I was unable to walk or talk. Therefore, I had to complete three weeks of intensive therapy (occupational, physical, and speech) as an in-patient. There were also months of in-home and outpatient therapy. First, I was wheelchair bound; then, I could use the walker. Finally in October 2006, I could walk with the cane only. Now, I seldom use the cane, but it's usually accessible, just in case I need it. Thanks to God, my husband, daughters, family, friends, physicians, hospital staff, and rehabilitation staff, I survived a life-or-death situation.

In the process of learning to deal with lupus, I have discovered a new calling: to increase lupus awareness and raise funds for research that would lead to better treatments and eventually a cure. When I was well enough, Cecil and I began volunteering with the Lupus Society of Illinois (LSI). In March 2010, we participated in the Lupus Foundation of America Advocacy Day. This is an annual event where interested parties from across the United States meet on Capitol Hill to help the members of Congress learn more about lupus, to discuss public policies which have an impact on people with lupus, and to encourage federal legislators to support more funding for lupus research and education.

LSI is a non-profit organization that "promotes lupus awareness and complements the work of healthcare professionals by providing personalized resources for the lupus community while supporting research." Cecil and I represent LSI at various area health fairs and local organizations. LSI also sponsors support groups throughout the state of Illinois. I served as group leader of their Hazel Crest lupus support group, now known as The Lupus Connection, for three years.

I also receive support, encouragement, and inspiration from

several other support groups: the Apostolic Church of God's Living Well With Lupus, Northwestern Hospital's Lupus in the Loop, and the Trinity United Church of God in Christ's lupus support group.

I also serve on two LSI-sponsored committees that help to raise funds to support lupus patients. One is the Southern Suburbs Lupus Walk Committee, which hosts an event in May (Lupus Awareness Month). Each year since its inception in 2009, my family and friends have worked hard so that our walk team, **K's Hope for a Cure**, can place among the top fundraisers in the Southern Suburbs Lupus Walk. I am also a member of the South Side Lupus Organization, which hosts the annual Holiday Dreams—Cure for Lupus Dinner Dance in December.

Today, I try to express gratitude for every day that I am alive and able to take care of myself. I still have painful and sore joints and find it difficult to walk sometimes. My voice is raspy, and I am not able to sing in the choir like I used to. I still have a mild productive cough, and I am easily fatigued. I forget or may not fully understand things at times. I second-guess most things I do.

Though my medication list is very long, I have developed a schedule that works well for me. I take calcium 500 mg +D three times a day stretched out over twenty-four hours and not within two hours of taking any other meds. That's a difficult one. My levothyroxine 100 mcg (thyroid hormone replacement) works best when taken on an empty stomach, so I take it when I first get up in the morning. After breakfast, I take a cocktail of: Plaquenil (hydroxychloroquine) 200 mg for lupus and potassium chloride 40 mEq to prevent low potassium levels; hydrochlorothiazide 12.5 mg, amlodipine 5 mg, losartan 25 mg, and metoprolol 100 mg for high blood pressure; and loratadine 10 mg and two sprays of azelastine HCL 0.1% 137 mg in each nostril for allergies. About one hour before dinner, I take pantoprazole 40 mg for gastroesophageal reflux disease (GERD). After dinner, I take another cocktail of Plaquenil 200 mg, potassium chloride 40 mEq, and vitamin D 1000 IU. Then before bed, I place one drop of latanoprost 0.005% in my left eye to maintain pressure, lubricant drops in my right eye for dryness, and I take pravastatin 10 mg to help control my cholesterol.

I am usually good about managing my stress by maintaining a schedule that incorporates regular exercise, relaxation, and meditation. I attend line dance classes for one hour on Monday and two hours on Thursday. On Tuesday, I complete forty-five minutes of Silver Pilates and fifty-five minutes of Aqua Aerobics. I ride a stationary bike for fifty minutes and work out on the UBE (upper body ergometer) machine for fifteen minutes on Wednesday. I try to do my sixty-minute at-home physical therapy routine on Friday, especially if I've missed the Wednesday bike session. If my energy level is low, I might just go to the gym and walk around the track a few times. At the very least, I try to do some form of exercise or movement thirty minutes a day, four days a week.

Most mornings, I meditate by spending time reading inspirational materials. I follow the Thru the Bible Radio Network schedule where we read the whole Bible over a five-year period. I also read from The One Year Chronological Bible. This time is also used to study my Sunday school lessons and to review the Daily Devotional issued by the New Faith Baptist Church International.

I awake each day being thankful to God for three main reasons: I am still alive; I can usually function independently; and I have loving, caring family members and friends who support me. A typical day for me goes like this: I have my prayer of thanks; I have my coffee and meditate; I eat my breakfast and take my morning medicines; I take other medications throughout the day and before going to bed; and I exercise or do physical therapy. Then, depending on my energy level, I complete my one big activity for the day. That activity may be a doctor's appointment, Bible study, church service, New Faith Seniors on The Move meeting, New Faith Health Care Ministry activity, vanity treatment (massage, facial, pedicure, or manicure), retirement group meeting, support group meeting, family reunion meeting, exercise class, bridge class, line dance class, a special function, or just reading and writing.

Yes, lupus is an incurable and life-threatening disease. The symptoms vary. The diagnosis is often very difficult to obtain. One never knows when a flare might occur. The treatments range from a few doctor's visits and medications to in-patient health care. The prognosis can range from fairly good health to death. Thank God that today, my condition is stable. So far, I am LIVING WELL WITH LUPUS.

Mom, the MV, and Me
(Unforgettable Circumstance)

**by Carla Y. Moore,
MS, CCC-SLP**

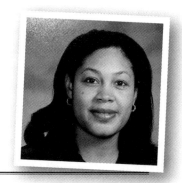

My mother retired in 2004 after working many years in education. For years she had suffered with annoying and unexplained symptoms such as fatigue, weight loss, and skin and scalp discoloration, and she had seen several specialists. She finally received the lupus diagnosis in February 2006. Unfortunately, before she was able to begin treatment, she suddenly began producing a bloody substance while coughing. She also experienced pains with each breath and swelling in her face. Fear pushed her to the emergency room, and that ended in a long stay in the intensive care unit at a local teaching hospital.

While in the ER, Mom's symptoms worsened, and the attending physician decided to keep her due to an abnormal cardiac report. That same night, my husband and I visited her in her hospital room. When visiting hours were over, we left. My mother appeared to be just fine. However, later that night, the physician on call ordered heparin, I guess, to regulate any blood clots. It is possible that the dosage increased the amount of blood and caused her heart to pump harder. She began experiencing cardiac arrest.

Approximately 7:00 a.m. the next morning, my step-father (Pops to me) called to tell me that Mom took a turn for the worse.

Some time during that night, she was sent to the surgery room to receive mechanical ventilation (MV) attention. When I arrived at the hospital, I learned that the pulmonary specialist could not locate the origin of bleeding. I stared at the monitor showing the video of pulmonary probe observation. Her capillaries appeared to be a collage of bloody strings. After tracheal intubation, which is the placement of a flexible plastic tube into the trachea (windpipe) to maintain an open airway, my mother was sent to the ICU and remained there for over two months.

During her stay in the ICU, Mom received chemotherapy. She couldn't talk due to the tracheal intubation, so I had to guess everything that she wanted to say to me. She heard the physician say that she needed chemotherapy, and that caused her grave concern. I figured out very fast that she wanted to know if she had cancer. I had to do a lot of explaining at that point. I said, "You see, in addition to corticosteroids, lupus can be treated with non-steroidal anti-inflammatory drugs, anti-malarial medications, and chemotherapy drugs." She did not buy that explanation. So, I just blurted out, "You ain't got cancer. Hear?" She appeared to be comfortable with that explanation.

Eventually, I realized that Mom needed a way to communicate with the hospital staff while I was not present. It was necessary for me to separate myself from being her daughter and wear my speech pathologist hat. I decided to use one of my new assistive technology devices, a portable keyboard, to allow her to type her thoughts. She was also encouraged to write down her thoughts on a tablet. After experiencing that whole chemotherapy episode, I was glad that she still had enough motivation to continue to communicate with others.

Shortly after the first few chemotherapy treatments, the hospital staff and our family began to encourage my mother to breathe independently of the ventilator. Even though there were days that I thought my mother was not going to ever breathe on her own, we continued to live our lives as if she was going to pull through this unforgettable circumstance. At one point, Pops and I felt that, perhaps, she needed someone from the psychiatric department to assist her with the weaning process. As a result, she was assessed and prescribed an antidepressant.

However, this was not a very good idea because the medication made her sleep too much, so she was not alert enough to sustain the test of breathing without the ventilator. We began to try other methods to assist with the weaning process. Pops arranged for her favorite television programs to coincide with the testing period. He would report to the ICU as though he was going to work at the bank, but he did not keep bankers' hours. He arrived very early and stayed very late. He would even stay all night at times. Almost daily, I would bring him dinner. I watched him rub her feet with lotion. He would help her with range of motion exercises. I even saw him cry for the first time. Our relationship became closer than ever before. We tried to continue our traditional events such as celebrating her birthday while she was taking the weaning test. Since Mom and Pops were in the process of having their house built, I brought decorating magazines for her to read during the testing period. At one point, we were contemplating placing my mother in a rehabilitation center that specializes in weaning from mechanical ventilators. After

> **"During her stay in the ICU, Mom received chemotherapy. She couldn't talk due to the tracheal intubation, so I had to guess everything that she wanted to say to me . . . Eventually, I realized that Mom needed a way to communicate with the hospital staff while I was not present . . . I decided to use one of my new assistive technology devices, a portable keyboard, to allow her to type her thoughts. She was also encouraged to write down her thoughts on a tablet."**

each visit, we would report our findings to her. She did not want to hear anything that we had to say. She did not look too happy about going to what she would call a nursing home. Although she couldn't talk, she made it known that she absolutely did not want to go to a nursing home. I guess the thought of that happening made her gradually breathe independently.

During the month of April, Mom finally passed the test that showed she was able to breathe on her own. However, as a result of being in the ICU for such a long period of time, she was not able to walk. Also, due to the extended length of time on the MV, she acquired aphonia (inability to produce voice). So Pops requested that the social worker seek availability at the Rehabilitation Institute of Chicago (RIC). While in RIC, she received occupational, physical, and speech therapy. After about a month in RIC, physical and speech therapies continued at home. Now, even after months of therapy, she still presents with difficulty in speaking, usually evidenced by a whispered hoarseness.

From Anger and Confusion to Understanding

by Celia Mimms, DDS

It was a Tuesday afternoon when I looked at my messages on my cell after class. My dad, who is not one to text but will leave a voicemail just to remind you to buy milk, had left a voicemail telling me to call him. I called back right away. The tone of his voice sounded distant and almost silent, but words still came through the line. He mentioned, "Your mother is in the hospital. You know she has been sick for a while."

I asked if I needed to leave school and come to the hospital, but he instantly replied, "No, just wait until the weekend." I wanted details, but he said that he would rather wait to tell me in person. It was like he was telling me this information so that I wouldn't hear it from anyone else first, but he didn't want me to worry.

So that Friday after my last class, I drove my usual three-hour route from Iowa City, Iowa, to Chicago, Illinois. My mind was racing as I was cruising along Interstate 80 like it was a motor speedway. All kinds of thoughts were bouncing inside my brain. *Why is she still in the hospital? Why can't I talk to her on the phone? Why is everyone so secretive about what is going on? Are they waiting on me to make life decisions? Does she have cancer? No, that can't be because the tests were all negative. Well medicine is not an exact science; sometimes they miss things. Could they have mixed up the results? What exactly is going on?*

By the time I arrived that night, it was too late to visit the hospital. My father assured me we would go first thing in the morning.

That night the house was eerily quiet. It was one of the most restless nights I ever had. I peeked into my father's room to see pillows in a straight line imitating my mother's body in the bed. *How long had this been going on, and why am I out of the loop?*

The next morning I waited for my father to wake up to go to the hospital. On the ride to downtown Chicago, he finally started talking.

"So, you know your mother has been sick for a while," he said. "Well, when you go down there, you will see a different side. She's *really* sick."

"Well how long do you think she will be in the hospital?" I asked.

There was a long pause.

"I really don't know." He paused again. "But don't let it scare you. She is improving."

We checked in and got on the elevator to floor 9—Intensive Care Unit (ICU). I stepped off the elevator to a rhythmic cadence of beeps, whistles of air, and a humming of machines. I walked into the room and saw an unconscious Black woman with tubes and wires extending from every part of her body. *This is not my mother; we are in the wrong room; she doesn't even know I'm in here. This is "improvement?"*

I didn't understand what was going on. I learned a little more later that day when my dad and I talked about Mom's condition. The term lupus came up. I learned more about how sick my mother was. I learned that without life support, my mother would not exist. Other family members came through that day, and it felt more like a funeral with people coming to "view the body."

I replayed the past twelve months in my head during the quiet times I was there in the room. How did my mother go from being active, working out regularly, cooking, etc., to a lifeless form that couldn't breathe without a machine? She was the one who was constantly on the move. Now, she had to communicate by answering yes-and-no questions with one versus two blinks. The last time I heard my mother's voice, we were fussing about something dumb. I didn't know that she would deteriorate to the point where she would never completely have her normal voice again.

For eleven weeks, I hid from people in Iowa the fact that my mother was even sick, let alone in ICU all of that time. Despite being mentally anguished during that time, I ended up getting my best grades in school. Spending weekends in the hospital around the medical community actually inspired me to pursue a career as a health care provider. I saw first-hand the impact that nurses, doctors, speech pathologists, occupational and physical therapists, and social workers had on families. The whole interworking of the hospital fascinated me. It was my second home for months.

There was just one issue: I didn't know what lupus was. The only face I saw was extreme pain and fatigue and that it could debilitate a person in an instant. I would read articles in journals and online, and they would focus on the two extremes. A person suffering from lupus either only had skin lesions or they had renal failure. There seemed to be no in-between; there was no cure, and everybody was going to die.

My mother survived her flare-up, had the smoothest, clearest skin that others envied, and did not have any kidney disorders. I figured the doctors diagnosed incorrectly once again. It was not until I was in dental school that I began to gain a more accurate understanding of lupus. After my comprehensive dental school training and my work as a dentist, I now know that everyone is affected differently, even within the oral cavity.

The Gold Medal Advocate

by Cecil Mimms, Jr.

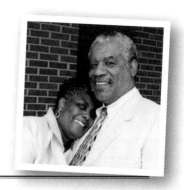

Iwatched as my wife started to have less energy and suffer more joint and muscle pain. It was really bad on Christmas Day 2005. As we prepared dinner for our large family gathering at our house, she said she needed to take a nap. Five or six hours later, she woke up to discover that everybody had finished eating and were almost ready to leave. She had slept through it all. That's when I knew she was *really* ill. They have an expression about lupus patients, "But you don't look sick." That was my wife, Kay.

For years, Kay tried to get explanations as to why she was always so tired and why her body hurt so much. She saw several medical professionals who treated the symptoms, but they were unable to provide a definite diagnosis. One of the specialists even performed a very painful bone marrow test for cancer. It was negative.

In January 2006, I called my cousin, Dr. Alfred Cook, who had graduated from and completed his internship at the Feinberg School of Medicine at Northwestern University. After we described Kay's symptoms, he recommended that we see Dr. Michael Zielinski, an internist who seemed to address medical mysteries and challenges with great enthusiasm. I think I was told that he loves to solve medical puzzles. We gathered all of Kay's medical records and took them with us for our first appointment with Dr. Zielinski. At the end of our appointment, he gained our confidence by looking into Kay's eyes and saying, "We are going to find out what's wrong with you."

After about two weeks Dr. Zielinski called and told us that he thought she had sarcoidosis, but he wanted to do one more test. After reviewing the additional test results, he gave us a definite diagnosis: lupus. Kay knew about two nieces who died from lupus. We suspected that there were other family members who suffered from the disease as well. Even though it was not what we wanted to hear, it was good to know the name and nature of the illness that had caused her so much suffering over the years.

We scheduled an appointment with Dr. Rosalind Ramsey-Goldman for Tuesday, February 14, at Northwestern. Dr. Ramsey-Goldman is an esteemed lupus researcher and rheumatologist who is noted for examining ways to improve the quality of life for people with lupus. We were now going to get treatment for this disease. Being diagnosed with lupus was a real shocker, but I felt confident that now Kay was going to get better. On the Sunday before our appointment with Dr. Ramsey-Goldman, Kay was in a lot of pain and was coughing up traces of blood. She stayed in the bed all day in a ball. That Monday morning, I told her we were going to the emergency room at Northwestern. I did not want to wait until the next day to see Dr. Ramsey-Goldman. When we arrived at the ER, we only waited a short while before they took us to an examining room. After running a few tests, they noticed she had some heart issues in addition to the muscle and joint pain she was experiencing. The ER doctors gave her something for the pain. Whatever it was knocked out the pain, and she felt better. In fact, she said she hadn't felt that good in a very long time. The concerns for the heart issues prompted them to admit her for further study of both the heart and lupus.

Later that evening, she had dinner and was feeling a lot better. Since she felt better, Kay suggested I go ahead with my plans to play tennis, and she would see me in the morning. Then about 11:30 p.m., I got a call from the hospital. They told me that she had started to leak blood from her lungs and was now in the cardiac section of the intensive care unit.

When I got to the ICU, Kay was sedated and on a breathing tube. Things had gone from having a good dinner and having no pain to seeing her this way. Things didn't seem promising to me.

Later that morning, the doctors made their rounds and gave me an update on what they had done overnight. The tube was put in to help Kay breathe easier. The monitors were recording her heartbeat, oxygen levels, blood pressure, breathing rate and pulse rate. The doctors were not sure at what point and why her lungs were bleeding. It was later deduced that the heparin given to reduce stress on the heart resulted in thinning her blood. The thinned blood was able to seep out because the lung walls had been weakened due to the effects of lupus. The plan was to take her off the propofol during their rounds so that she could respond to their questions.

That night and the next couple of days I stayed in the ICU room.

Even though it was not customary, the nurses brought in a cot for me. During the day, the doctors would make their rounds. After doing a test where they looked into the lungs to see if there was any damaged tissue, they determined Kay was getting better. The lungs were no longer seeping blood. My cousin, Dr. Cook, stopped by that Thursday and encouraged me concerning Kay's condition. He thought she seemed to be doing pretty good considering what she had been through.

The plan was that Kay might go home the next day. Later that night a new night nurse came on duty and told me I couldn't stay in the ICU overnight. At about 8:30 p.m. as I was preparing to go home, all of Kay's vital signs started to go haywire. I called the nurse and yelled, "Get in here right now." Kay's heart was racing. Her blood pressure was all over the chart. They called a code blue. They worked on her for a couple of hours and finally got her stable around 11:00 p.m.

I went home that night, but I was back at 7:00 a.m. the next morning. She was still stable; however, the doctors were still concerned as to why her vitals fluctuated so much the night before. I was asked to sign consent forms for a blood transfusion because of the blood she had lost the day before.

The doctors also wanted to do an angiogram to see if there was any damage to the heart. They explained that during the procedure, it was customary to use blood thinners. They explained further that if they found damage or clots, they would normally put in a stent. The procedure might cause excessive bleeding. They were cautious because they felt that if Kay started to bleed during the procedure, they might not be able to stop the bleeding, and she would bleed out. The attending doctors consulted with the cardiac and pulmonary specialists to help in making a decision about the best course of action. It was later decided to do the angiogram for discovery only. If they found anything, they would know the extent of the damage but would not do anything at that time. The test results showed that there was no blockage.

The doctors decided that Kay's main issues now were with the lungs and not so much with the heart. They felt resolution of her issues could be handled better in the pulmonary ICU. So they moved her out of the cardiac ICU. They also explained that since using propofol as a sedative was intended for short periods, they were replacing it with another sedative. With the new sedative, she would be more alert. They also put in a tracheotomy tube.

Over the next sixty days, I was at the hospital from 7:00 a.m. until 9:00 p.m. every day. The nurses worked twelve-hour shifts, from 8:00 to 8:00. Before I left at night, I met the night nurse and let her know who I was. In the mornings, I checked with the night nurse again to get a report about what happened overnight. Then I greeted the day nurse and discussed the plans for the day. The day/night ritual went on the entire time Kay was in the ICU.

During the first week in the pulmonary ICU, doctors from the cardiac team, the pulmonary team, and the rheumatology team saw Kay daily. At first they just checked her vital signs and read the nurses reports. By the second week, Kay was starting to get stronger. The doctors decided to reduce her medications just

"Over the next sixty days, I was at the hospital from 7:00 a.m. until 9:00 p.m. every day. The nurses worked twelve-hour shifts, from 8:00 to 8:00 ... In the mornings, I checked with the night nurse ... to get a report about what happened overnight. Then I greeted the day nurse and discussed the plans for the day. The day/night ritual went on the entire time {my wife} was in the ICU ... The one thing that we did each morning ... was to greet each other with a wink and a smile. When I got my wink and smile, I knew she had a good night. Then I would talk with the nurse."

before they came by, so that she could start to participate in the daily rounds by nodding. Our older daughter, Carla, brought in one of her communication picture charts. That allowed Kay to answer questions by pointing to pictures on the chart. There was not a lot of communication going on because Kay was still sedated and slept a lot.

The one thing that we did each morning when I got there was to greet each other with a wink and a smile. When I got my wink and smile, I knew she had had a good night. Then I would talk with the nurse.

Kay was not breathing on her own, so she was on a respirator. Mucus would build up in her tracheotomy tube, and then the respiratory therapist would have to come in to clean it. This process needed to be done about every two hours.

Kay was in a room that was designed for patients with infectious diseases. It had a separate entrance through what they called a clean room, but that entrance was never used. Kay's room had only one patient bed with two chairs, a nurse's desk with a monitor, and a restroom. The room had a large sliding glass door that stayed open all day until 10:00 p.m. and was reopened at 7:00 a.m. Housekeeping cleaned the room each morning. The bed linen was changed by the night nurse. The night nurse also bathed and changed the patient. While in the ICU, Kay's room had two trees of IV pumps. One tree was used just for glucose and sedatives; the other tree was used to dispense various medications. There was a monitor that displayed heart rhythms, blood pressure, oxygen levels, and breathing rate. Since I was there all the time, I started to know how to read the monitors and notice the differences in sounds from the respirator. If the monitoring center did not respond to changes right away, I would call the nurse and let them know that something needed their attention.

The hospital staff wore unique uniform colors that were assigned by the duties they performed. This helped patients and their family members to recognize and identify which healthcare department was interacting with them. I learned the colors of the clothing the hospital staff wore:

- white short jackets—medical students
- white long coats (no patches)—interns
- white long coats (with patches)—attending
- gray long coats—residents, department heads
- light green/gray scrubs—doctors

- light blue scrubs—nurses
- dark green scrubs—physical, occupational, respiratory therapists; radiology
- dark blue scrubs—housekeeping

This was very helpful to me as I met different medical staff coming in to do different procedures.

During the second week in the pulmonary ICU, Kay improved, and they started to address the lupus. They sent bloodwork out to a lab in California to determine the type of lupus she had and what her white blood cell levels were. They also monitored the white blood cells in Northwestern. The levels were extremely high, so they scheduled her first set of chemotherapy treatments of Cytoxan. When they gave it to her, it made her very nauseated.

Possibly in anticipation of and preparation for removal of the

> **"As we moved into the third week, Kay continued to improve. When the doctors made their rounds, she was more involved in her treatment. I had learned to read Kay's lips and understand what she wanted. When we talked to the doctors ... Kay would mouth the responses to me, and I would tell the doctors what she said. Sometimes I would get it wrong, but she would repeat it until I got it right. We were a good team."**

feeding tube, the dietician started Kay on a liquid diet. This caused her to produce a loose stool. That required frequent changes of clothing for the patient and linen for the bed. One of the nurses tried to help Kay feel less embarrassed about the inability to control her bowel movements. He would try to make her laugh about her condition by saying things like, "Oops, clean up on aisle six", or "Are you in pain? I have drugs." He also introduced us to a product that worked sort of like a urine catheter but used at the other end (rectum). He called it the Zazzy. This stopped the frequent changes to the patient and bedding.

As we moved into the third week, Kay continued to improve. When the doctors made their rounds, she was more involved in her treatment. I had learned to read Kay's lips and understand what she wanted. When we talked to the doctors, they would ask Kay how she felt, what hurt, what she needed, and if she had any questions. Kay would mouth the responses to me, and I would tell the doctors what she said. Sometimes I would get it wrong, but she would repeat it until I got it right. We were a good team.

Kay developed an infection, and this set her progress back a little. She fought through it and started to get stronger. She was able to move her arms and feet, and we worked on her finger movement. This prompted the ICU staff to place an order for her to have occupational and physical therapy in her room. They told us that normally they didn't do therapy in the ICU, but they made an exception because she was doing so well.

The major issues keeping her in the ICU revolved around the feeding tube, muscle weakness, and being on the respirator. The speech therapy department performed an evaluation and determined the feeding tube could be removed. One down; two to go.

As she started to eat soft food, her strength improved. Two down; one to go. The last one was the toughest. Kay had been on the respirator for so long that she had become dependent on it. She didn't need it, but it was hard for her to let go. That was a battle. Kay said that when off the respirator, it felt like she was breathing through a straw. The more we tried to get her off, the deeper she dug in her heels. We wanted her off that machine so that she could be accepted at the Rehabilitation Institute of Chicago (RIC). The RIC did not accept patients who were on a respirator.

The hospital was now saying that she had to leave because she was stable, and the room was needed. I told them, "Don't give me that BS." But we knew the time would come when Kay would have to leave, even if it meant going to a long-term care facility. Carla and I then started researching and visiting rehabilitation centers that were successful at removing patients from respirators and accepted our health insurance. One of the doctors had done his residency with my cousin and recommended a place in Hinsdale. Carla and I went to see it. It was a nice place. It used to be a tuberculosis sanitarium in the '50s and early '60's. We felt it was a good option, but the insurance would not cover charges at that facility. Two other places were suggested to us, one on North Sheridan Road in Chicago, and one in Indiana. After our visits, we both decided that the Indiana facility would be a good choice.

The time came when we had to leave Northwestern and go to the rehab center to be weaned from the vent. The day before we were to leave, they did another test to wean Kay off the respirator, something we did just about every day. The respiratory therapist came in and told Kay he would be starting the test. (What he meant was the test would be starting soon. But Kay thought he meant he was actually starting the test then.) When they came to start the test, Kay hit the ceiling. She said in her way of communicating, "What are you talking about? I have already been on the test for an hour." She was very angry because she felt that she had wasted a lot of time trying to breath without the machine and now knew there was no way she could last the eight hours that were needed to pass the test. We tried to explain that the test was starting now. She got so mad that she said, "Just forget it," and decided she wasn't going back on the respirator. Her stubbornness proved to be what we needed to get her off the respirator. We were then able to cancel the rehab center in Indiana, and we moved her to a regular hospital room.

Kay stayed in the regular room for about a week. At first, she was placed in a nice big room at the end of the hall. I spent the first night with her but went home the second night. She had a really bad night. She experienced extreme cold, and her joint pain worsened. She still could not walk or talk. I guess that was not considered when they assigned her a room so far from the nurse's station. So when she buzzed and the nurses asked her what she needed, they could not hear her response. After three days in the regular room, they moved her to a room across from the nurse's station.

Each day, Kay received a breathing treatment administered by the respiratory therapist (RT). She also received occupational therapy (OT), physical therapy (PT), and speech therapy (ST).

Even though the hospital staff thought that she was not strong enough to go to RIC, she passed their evaluation and was accepted. This was great news. So as soon as a bed was open, we moved her to RIC. We just unplugged everything and whisked her through the underground passage that goes from Northwestern to RIC. We didn't want that opening to get away or have RIC reverse their decision.

Kay's therapy sessions at RIC were very intense. The nurses administered medications throughout the day, the OT supervised the hygiene and dress, and the PT helped Kay complete individual sessions in the therapy gym. Later in the day the OT assistant would lead the group therapy session. There were also individual sessions with the ST. At the end of the day, Kay would be exhausted.

There was one day when it was time for Kay's afternoon OT group class. She was very tired and decided she could skip the OT class because she felt it was just baby stuff. She asked me to put her in the bed, and I did. Next thing we know, the OT assistant (privately we called her "the Sarge") came into the room, crawled into Kay's bed and said, "Oh no! You have to get out of there and go to therapy. You are never to miss a therapy session. You need this." The Sarge was small and short, but she pulled Kay out of the bed, sat her in the wheelchair, and pushed her to class. Kay never missed that class again. In fact, a lot of the times, the Sarge made me participate in the class too. She was a good person and helped everyone get stronger.

The therapists at RIC were very proficient. Kay worked very hard and started to progress quickly by working on completing her own hygiene routine, transferring from bed to wheelchair, getting in and out of cars, using a walker, and maneuvering on one or two steps. Sixty plus days prior, Kay had started this journey. After a month at RIC, it was time to go home and continue to improve.

At home, Kay received visits from the ST, the PT, and the nurse for thirty days. It was pretty hectic trying to keep up with who was coming and when. Using a big desk calendar was a big help. We still use it today to keep up with all of our activities.

"'Oh no! You have to get out of {bed} and go to therapy. You are never to miss a therapy session. You need this.' The Sarge was small and short, but she pulled Kay out of the bed, sat her in the wheelchair, and pushed her to class. Kay never missed that class again. In fact, a lot of the times, the Sarge made me participate in the class too. She was a good person and helped everyone get stronger."

After the at-home therapy, we started outpatient therapy at RIC in Homewood. While at home, every night I had to flush Kay's PICC line (a long, thin, flexible tube that was inserted in her arm and used to give medicines over a long period of time). I kind of looked forward to it. I think Kay did too. This became a special time and bond between us.

Now Kay is doing very well. She takes a lot of medications and has some limitations, but we are grateful that she is alive and that we can bond in more enjoyable ways.

Postscript by Kay Mimms

Cecil has written about a few of the ways he served as my advocate during the three months that I was in the hospital and rehab. I want to share some examples that stand out for me.

Cecil came to the hospital and rehab every day and sometimes stayed overnight. The few times he needed to be away, he would have one of my friends stay with me. I overheard one of the doctors say, "I've never been in this room when he wasn't here."

Since Cecil was at the hospital a lot, he established a great relationship with the doctors, nurses, therapists, and other hospital staff. He kept detailed records of procedures, explanations, plans, and even a list with the names of the medical staff members who provided services for me. He learned the rules, regulations, and even the dress code of the hospital staff. When he approached them with questions and concerns, he could address them by name. Then, they were more willing to provide the information and advice he needed. He earned the sympathy and respect of the hospital staff, so I suspect they went the extra mile to provide us with inside information.

Cecil accompanied me to my doctor's appointments and therapy sessions, even after I regained driving privileges. He even participated in some of my group therapy sessions.

Because he wanted me to receive rehab at the best facility possible, Cecil tried to think of all kinds of things that would motivate me to come off the ventilator. He stood up to those who recommended that I be moved to a facility with fewer opportunities for rapid progress. In fact, he made sure I received services, sometimes unusual ones like OT and PT in the ICU, until he was satisfied that I was stable enough to be moved to a different area in the hospital or a different facility altogether. In general, he was determined that I receive the best care possible.

Cecil has called me his Virginia Slims Baby ("You've come a long way, baby"). If I were a judge on the Lupus Olympic Committee, I would call him the **Gold Medal Advocate.**

Quite the Lupus Survivor

by Michael Zielinski, MD, FACP

In order to help me piece together and get a clearer understanding of my lupus journey, I asked my primary care physician, Dr. Michael D. Zielinski, to write about his impressions. He was gracious enough to share some of his thoughts and feelings. This is a synopsis of his review.

There are some initial patient encounters that you do not forget, and Kay was one of those. As a primary care doctor, one of the skills you learn with experience is how to identify when someone is sick, and it was clear that Kay was sick.

Kay was referred to me by her cousin, whom I had met while he was training to become a doctor. She had not felt well for a few months and had a long list of symptoms. She complained of losing weight, fatigue, achiness, and being more out of breath at times. She had seen other doctors and thankfully brought in her extensive workup. In addition to her worrisome symptoms, there were a few things that initially convinced me that something *big* was up.

During the exam, I noted a few locations where her lymph glands were swollen. Her blood work revealed that all of her major blood cells were low--that is, her white cells (which fight infection), her red cells (which transport oxygen), and her platelets (clotting cells). Interestingly, she had had a bone marrow biopsy for the workup of this, and it appeared her bone marrow was working well. That made a diagnosis of lymphoma, or even leukemia, much less likely.

Once I examined her and asked her all of my questions, I sent her for a few more blood tests and a chest x-ray. My initial thought was that she might have sarcoidosis, a disease that is more common in African Americans and that can definitely result in a lot of symptoms and blood abnormalities. I also ordered an antinuclear antibody or ANA test to see if there is any "autoimmune" process going on. That would cover checking for most diseases where essentially the body is attacking itself.

A few days later when I received the lab results, I noted that her ANA test was through the roof and in a pattern consistent with lupus. All of her symptoms would be explained by this diagnosis. I had taken care of patients with lupus before, mostly while I was in training, but this was the first time I was the one making the diagnosis. I remembered having the good fortune of working with Dr. Ramsey-Goldman, our local and nationally known lupus expert. It was a wonderful training and allowed me to see a wide variety of lupus patients with her. There were patients who were quite ill with multiple complications and others who had their disease under control. Now that I had the diagnosis for Kay, I knew our lupus specialist would be the right doctor for her to see. I gave Kay the initial information and told her to arrange an appointment as soon as possible.

One of the unfortunate aspects of being a good doctor is that your schedule is always booked. Kay called me back saying that it was going to be a few weeks before she could get an appointment with Dr. Ramsey-Goldman. I told Kay to keep in touch with me in terms of her symptoms. But it was frustrating that I was unable to get Kay in for treatment as soon as I would have liked. If I remember correctly, the day before Kay was to have seen Dr. Ramsey-Goldman, I received a call that she had increased chest pains and shortness of breath. She came to the emergency room and was admitted to the hospital. Then she started coughing up blood and was found to have a hemorrhage in her lungs. She ended up intubated on a ventilator. Frankly, I felt horrible when I heard about this, and I wondered if Kay's ICU experience could have been prevented had she been able to have the lupus treated sooner.

Because our hospital has a hospitalist system in which admitted patients are only seen by physicians who work exclusively in that facility, I was not Kay's primary attending physician during her stay. However, I did receive calls and updates from the hospital doctors on a regular basis. When you are in the hospital that

> **"As a primary care doctor, it's hard, yet quite rewarding and challenging in a good way, to take care of patients with rheumatologic disorders like lupus because: a) it affects nearly every organ system, and b) just about everybody has multiple symptoms that need to be waded through. Certain symptoms can be followed, whereas, other ones need to be looked into and treated aggressively. Kay has been one of the lucky ones."**

long, complications happen on a routine basis. Therefore, it's not uncommon that Kay developed heart rhythm issues, blood clots, gastritis, infections, muscle weakness, you name it. With that being said, she fought off all of these issues and came back to see me in my office about three months after her initial diagnosis. She was clearly tired and beat up, but I was really happy to see her out of the hospital. She had had a stay at the Rehabilitation Institute of Chicago. They really set her on the right path.

Over the next year or so, I was busy following up mostly on the complications she had from her hospitalization. She was also followed closely by rheumatologists, started on Plaquenil, and was on a tapering dose of prednisone to help keep her lupus in check. She showed some improvement with each visit.

Over the past few years, Kay has become quite the survivor with lupus, with no big flares since the initial one in 2006. There are certain things that have really never returned to normal for Kay since the hospitalization, but overall it has been great for me to see her recover and live as normal of a life as possible.

As a primary care doctor, it's hard, yet quite rewarding and challenging in a good way, to take care of patients with rheumatologic disorders like lupus because: a) it affects nearly every organ system, and b) just about everybody has multiple symptoms that need to be waded through. Certain symptoms can be followed, whereas, other ones need to be looked into and treated aggressively. Kay has been one of the lucky ones. She's had great care from her rheumatologist, and luckily her disease has responded to a fairly safe and easy-to-take medication like Plaquenil. I hope her disease course follows this pattern for a very long time.

A Physician's Perspective

by Rosalind Ramsey-Goldman, MD, DrPH
Solovy Arthritis Research Society
Research Professor of Medicine/Rheumatology

Part 1: The Elusive Enemy (Mimms)

Although the idea of a warm weather vacation sounded good, it likely precipitated the lupus flare because sun exposure is a known trigger of SLE. The primary care physician is one of the first health care providers who may see a patient who might have SLE. The diagnosis can be missed unless the doctor thinks that it might be SLE. It is important to teach all health care providers who are on the front lines to be familiar with this disease so they can initiate the process of making a correct diagnosis.

Teaching Point: Lupus is hard to diagnose; sun exposure can precipitate a flare.

Part 1: The Wake (Mimms)

The patient was sedated, and her breathing was assisted with machines. SLE was also being treated with high-dose steroids which can also distort thinking. Finally, she also needed to be resuscitated with the "bolt of electricity" because her heart stopped beating. This is a striking description of what it felt like from the patient's perspective.

Teaching Point: Problems related to lupus can be serious, including difficulty breathing or heartbeat abnormalities.

Part 2: Lupus Does Not Have Me (Fields)

The skin is one of the common areas affected by lupus. The skin graft referred to in this chapter is really a skin biopsy, which is a test in which a small piece of skin is removed and studied under the microscope. This type of test helps doctors know if the skin rash might be caused by SLE. Again, a combination of symptoms and test results which can be from the blood, urine, or skin in this case, are used to make a diagnosis of SLE. Once the diagnosis is made, the patient can have difficulty accepting this answer. Support and motivation help someone cope with a chronic illness like SLE.

Teaching Point: Learn as much as you can about the disease. Knowledge can be empowering.

Part 2: My Time is Coming (Rias)

Pregnancy, when lupus is active, can be difficult. Babies may be born early and be too small. However, with specialized care, these tiny infants can survive. Planning pregnancy when you have lupus is critical since many specialists may need to be involved to treat both mother and child in order to have a good outcome for both patients. Ask questions and try to learn as much as you can about lupus and how it is affecting you.

Teaching Point: Pregnancy planning is needed between the patient/family and the treating physician for the best outcome for mother and baby.

Part 2: A Strong Family (Sanders)

It can take several years and many doctor visits before the correct diagnosis is made. Unfortunately lupus can progress rapidly in some individuals. The kidney becomes scarred and can no longer function, and the patient needs dialysis to clean the body of its waste. Although there is a genetic or familial pre-disposition to develop lupus, families may have only one affected member or several affected members. There is ongoing research to understand how genetics predisposes someone to develop lupus or to get severe lupus.

Teaching Point: Lupus is hard to diagnose. Research is needed to understand the genetic predisposition to lupus so we can work on preventing damage from the disease and ideally preventing it from occurring in the first place.

Part 2: Shaking out the Cobwebs (Burleson)

In the early 1950s, the main medication used to treat lupus was steroids, including adrenocorticotropic hormone (ACTH) treatments and cortisone. Lupus can go into remission and be quiet for many years. Pregnancy outcomes are most favorable during the time when lupus is not active. As people age, they can develop other problems such as polymyalgia rheumatica, which is not related to lupus even though it is often also treated with steroids like prednisone.

Teaching Point: Lupus treatment has come a long way since the 1950s, but we still have a long way to go. Research is needed to bridge this gap in knowledge.

Part 3: Shining the Light on Lupus (Chappell-Rice)

It can take a long time before someone gets a diagnosis of lupus. You can look well, but on the inside, lupus can be causing problems and unexplained symptoms like fatigue or pain—symptoms that are hard to see or measure with a test. Pregnancy, when lupus is not controlled, can be risky for both mother and baby. In this case, lupus became even more active during pregnancy and could even flare more after the pregnancy is over. In this case, the placenta separated from the womb too soon, resulting in blood loss which was life threatening for both mother and child. Unfortunately the baby did not survive, but this mother is strong and has found the will to live, the drive to improve lupus awareness, and the mission to highlight the importance of research because we need better treatments for lupus.

Teaching Points: There can be a delay in diagnosing lupus. Pregnancy can be difficult if lupus is not controlled prior to conceiving.

Part 3: My Lupus, My Faith, My Story (Rose)

Contrasting emotions such as denial, tenacity, faith, and acceptance are ways one might cope with chronic illness which led to dialysis and still being able to work on days when not on dialysis. Pregnancy while on dialysis is very high-risk. Babies born to mothers on dialysis are frequently born early and small, and they have many medical problems related to their preterm birth. Even with care in specialized neonatal intensive care units, the outcome may not be successful. There are many ways, such as being a foster parent, to fulfill the dream of parenthood.

Teaching Point: Women with lupus can be mothers, including through adoption and foster care. Sometimes you have to find another way to follow your dreams, and this is one example of learning how to cope.

Part 3: Advocate for Cure/Angels Standing Guard/Kind of Like the Huxtables (Collins Family)

Misdiagnosis occurs too often in SLE, especially in the setting of neurological problems. A chronic illness not only affects the patient, but all those closest to her or him. Support systems are essential in helping one deal with a life-threatening illness. Giving back, such as volunteering to help others with lupus, is another way to feel empowered when one is ill.

Teaching Points: Lupus is hard to diagnose, and misdiagnosis occurs too often. Support systems are needed to help individuals deal with chronic illness.

Part 3: Grateful for Life (Bryant)

One of the complications of having lupus is an increased risk of infection, so if you have an unexplained fever you should seek medical attention right away. If you are not certain what to do, then a second opinion should be sought. If lupus causes damage or complications, such as kidney failure or an infection destroying joints, there may be a negative impact on one's ability to do one's job, and one may lose insurance coverage or need to go on disability. One's support system helps one look to the future, even if it is different from what one envisioned for one's self.

Teaching Points: Having lupus can cause organ damage, and this can lead to the inability to work and the need to consider going on disability.

Part 3: Something Called Lupus (Carreón)

Ask questions about your diagnosis and the recommended

treatment. Even if the doctor has explained all of this, the patient may not understand the advice and not follow it. If the explanation is not clear, ask again. Even if you have lupus, you can have other medical problems such as diabetes, heart attacks, or cancer. It is important to have a positive attitude when you are challenged with health issues. Lupus can run in families, or someone can be the only one in the family who is affected by lupus.

Teaching Point: Lupus patients can have other medical conditions.

Part 3: My Lupie Bio (Spadoni)

Lupus can be difficult to diagnose, and once you know your diagnosis, find a doctor you trust on this life-long journey.

Teaching Point: Lupus can be hard to diagnose.

Part 3: Challenges to Remission: Hope for Removal (Douglas)

Kidney problems are the most common severe problem experienced by lupus patients. Treatments are usually effective but can have side effects which include infections, swelling, difficulty sleeping, fatigue, and pain.

Teaching Point: Research is needed to improve treatment for lupus. Our goal is discover more effective treatments that have fewer side effects.

Part 3: The Bullet That Hit the Lupus Target (Clark) Mental illness presents special challenges when other medical problems such as lupus occur. Lithium is one medication used to treat a mental illness called bipolar disorder. It can be very tricky to use, because it can be difficult to find the right dose for

a particular patient. If too little is given, then it does not work to manage the highs and lows of bipolar disorder. However, if the level of lithium is too high, then it can cause problems with the brain and kidneys, which could also be problems seen in other conditions such as lupus.

Teaching Point: Drugs have been implicated in a condition called drug-induced lupus, and when this situation occurs the symptoms of lupus resolve once the medication is stopped. If lupus continues, then the drug may have unmasked lupus or may not have been the reason lupus developed in the first place. All medications used should be monitored closely for side effects. In this case, lithium may or may not have caused lupus. We need more research to understand the difference between drug-induced lupus and systemic lupus.

Part 3: Resilient (Buford)

The diagnosis of lupus can be difficult to make because of the different symptoms that can occur all at once or over time. Also, most patients who have lupus are the only ones in their family with the disease.

Teaching Point: It is not unusual for family members to worry if they might develop lupus in the future. More research is needed to understand how genetics plays a role in someone's risk for developing lupus so we can work toward preventing it from happening at all.

Part 3: Navigating the Path Toward Health and Wellness (Mebane)

Increasing awareness about lupus is needed for both patients and health care providers. It is not unusual to have to see several doctors before the correct diagnosis is made.

Teaching Point: Lupus affects not only the patients but also their family members and friends.

Part 3: My Life with Lupus (Blessed: Not Broken) (Walker)

Daily activities can be difficult. Family members may notice that things have changed. You may look good but not feel well. Even health care providers may not recognize something is wrong. It is important to see a rheumatologist—a specialist who understands, diagnoses, and treats connective tissue and auto-immune disorders such as lupus. Medications treat symptoms, but they can have side effects. Helping others is one way of helping one's self.

Teaching Point: Getting encouragement from family, friends, and support groups is one way to cope with disease and take charge of your life when you have a chronic illness.

Part 4: The Latest Leg of My Journey (Lindsey)

Although anything can happen with lupus, it is important to realize that other medical problems can arise and will need specific treatment while you have lupus.

Teaching Point: Seek care when you do not know if lupus or something else is wrong. Learn how to be your own advocate for care.

Part 4: Armed with Hope & Knowledge (Ambler)

With lupus, kidney disease is the most common problem. A kidney specialist known as a nephrologist works closely with the rheumatologist to manage this serious problem and to monitor the medications used to treat it. Learning as much as you can helps your health care providers take care of you.

Teaching Point: Maintaining a healthy lifestyle by eating a nutritious diet, being physically active within your daily activities, and smoking cessation if you smoke cigarettes are essential parts of managing lupus. A healthy lifestyle will support the medical treatments you receive for lupus and help minimize organ damage.

Part 4: Living Well with Lupus (Mimms)/Mom, The MV and Me (Unforgettable Circumstance) (Moore)/The Gold Medal Advocate (Mimms)

This is another example where it took a long time to make the diagnosis of lupus even though the clues were there the whole time. Primary care physicians are frequently the first doctors to see patients with their initial symptoms. The key to getting the diagnosis right is for the physician to be aware of the many ways lupus can present, to think this might be the answer, and then refer the patient to a rheumatologist, who is experienced in confirming the diagnosis of lupus. Severe, life-threatening symptoms can suddenly occur, so some patients must be admitted to the hospital in order to get the treatment they need. Family and friend support and a positive attitude help deal with this chronic illness.

Teaching Point: Improved education of health care providers and availability of community services for patients help newly diagnosed patients and those with established disease manage their disease. Some organizations that help lupus patients by providing support, education, advocacy, and research services are described below.

- "The Lupus Research Institute (LRI) is uniquely dedicated to novel research in lupus."[42]
- "The Lupus Initiative is a national education program designed to reduce health disparities experienced by patients with lupus."[43]
- The Lupus Foundation of America (LFA) is "devoted to solving the mystery of lupus,...while giving caring support to those who suffer from its brutal impact."[44]
- The Lupus Society of Illinois (LSI) provides personal support to people living with lupus in Illinois. "As a member of the Lupus Research Institute (LRI) National Coalition we know the voice of Illinois' lupus community will be heard on a national level."[45]

Part 4: Quite the Lupus Survivor (Dr. Zielinski)

A well trained primary care physician is a critical partner with the rheumatologist to diagnose and manage the disease.

Part 5
Striving and Thriving in the Lupus Lane

Living My Best Life with Lupus

In their *Many Shades* lupus pamphlet, the NIH reports that there is no cure yet for lupus, but most cases can be managed if diagnosed in time (before organ involvement) and if properly treated.[46] The American College of Rheumatology offers four key tips for managing and living well with lupus: (1) form a solid support system of health care professionals, friends and family; (2) be involved with your treatment plan and educate yourself about lupus; (3) incorporate bouts of light to moderate activity into your daily routine when possible while respecting your body's need to rest in between; and (4) avoid excess sun exposure.[47]

Based on my own personal experiences and the recommendations I've received from my care team and other lupus patients, the following proactive steps have helped me to manage my lupus so far:

- Continuing to learn about lupus so that I get a better understanding of the disease and its potential impact on my life and the lives of those with whom I live.

- Actively participating in my own care. I also have an advocate, someone who accompanies me to doctor visits and helps me keep records of health information related to my journey with lupus.
- Searching for health care providers who are familiar with lupus and who will listen to and address my concerns.
- Scheduling regular checkups, instead of just when a concern arises.
- Following instructions for taking medications.
- Maintaining good communication with my health care team. Seeking information on all issues (use of sunscreen, stress management, structured exercise, rest, vaccinations, preventive health care, and care needed from other specialists such as cardiologists, dentists, dermatologists, ophthalmologists, nephrologists, neurologists, pharmacists, nurses, therapists, and so on).
- Always sharing accurate and complete medical information with my team of health care providers. Maintaining a detailed list of concerns and questions, and bringing my list, along with a copy for the doctor, to each office visit. My doctors have expressed that they like when I have my list because it makes it easier for them to see the whole picture. It also helps me to remember all that I want to discuss.

- Paying close attention to my body, mind, and spirit. Learning to recognize the warning signs of a flare and taking steps to prevent it or reduce its intensity. Possible warning signs for me include difficulty breathing, dizziness, hair loss, headaches, increased fatigue, more joint pain and stiffness, muscle aches, rashes or blisters, and swelling.

- Discussing any plans for treatment changes with my health care team.

- After discussion with my health care team, using appropriate stress management techniques such as exercise, relaxation, and meditation.

- Establishing realistic goals and priorities for managing my time and energy. Planning for adequate rest and quiet.

- Maintaining a good support system of family, friends, medical professionals, community organizations, faith-based groups and support groups.

- Staying involved in social activities as much as possible.

- Limiting the time I spend in the sun. Even though I hate wearing hats, I try to remember to wear one if I'm going to be outside for any length of time. I use sunscreen every day, even if I'm going to be inside.

- Trying to follow guidelines for a healthy diet.

Using Research as a Route Toward Improvement in Diagnostics and Treatment and Discovery of a Cure

"Lupus is one of the cruelest, most mysterious diseases on earth. It strikes without warning, has unpredictable and sometimes fatal effects, lasts a lifetime, and has no known cure."[48] "Fifty years ago, survival was 50 percent after four years. Today, thanks to advances brought about by research... it is 97 percent at five years and 90 percent at ten years."[49] Let's review a few of the contributions that have been and might be realized through research.

According to the NIH Handout, lupus research is a major focus at NIAMS. The program "sponsored the development of a Lupus Family Registry and Repository that gathers medical information, as well as blood and tissue samples from patients and their relatives."[50] Now, researchers all over the U.S. have access to this information. NIAMS also helped to establish a registry to collect information and blood samples from children affected by neonatal lupus and their mothers. This information is used to counsel families and to track data such as recurring rates in subsequent pregnancies. Other NIAMS research areas include genetics, biomarkers, disease process, treatment, and barriers that prevent certain populations from complying with their prescribed treatment plans.

Though the causes of lupus have not been discovered, many scientists report that heredity, hormones, and the environment must be involved.[51] "Evidence for the importance of genes in the etiology of human lupus has been provided by studies showing that 1) there is a higher concordance of lupus between identical twins than between fraternal twins; and 2) relatives of patients with lupus are at higher risk for developing the disease. A number of genes have been found in association with lupus in human populations... Because of the complexity and heterogeneity of lupus, however, researching the genes involved in the disease and its many features is laborious, time-consuming and expensive. To be successful, lupus gene discovery will require continued concentrated effort by many groups."[52]

"In studies of identical twins, when one twin has lupus, the other twin has a 24 percent chance of developing it. This and other research suggests that genetics plays an important role, but it also shows that genes alone do not determine who gets lupus, and that other factors play a role"[53]

"New ideas, concepts and technologies allow the study of how genes interact with each other and with the environment to cause disease in the predisposed individuals."[54]

Anyone, regardless of age, ethnic background, or socioeconomic status, can be diagnosed with lupus; however, it is most common in young women, and particularly those of African American, Asian, Hispanic/Latino, and Native American descent. "Women with the disease outnumber men 9 to 1. It often strikes women in their early working and childbearing years, interfering with the ability to work, have or raise a family or in some cases even care for themselves."[55]

"Because of their disease severity and young age, lupus is a particular burden for children. Thus, any research that leads to improved understanding, treatment and quality of life in children has significant, lifelong implications."[56] "Research on these high-risk populations is a major focus of lupus investigators."[57]

"The most heterogeneous of the autoimmune diseases, lupus is also one of the most difficult to understand and treat."[58] Treatment plans may include several medications and are tailored to the specific needs of the patient. NIH reports that in March 2011, the U.S. Food and Drug Administration approved the first new drug, Benlysta, for lupus patients in more than fifty years. "Studies have found that adding Benlysta to commonly used lupus medications can reduce lupus disease activity. In fact, in clinical trials, Benlysta plus other lupus treatments was superior to other lupus treatments alone in reducing lupus disease activity."[59] In two of three studies, fewer African Americans who received Benlysta responded to treatment compared to African Americans who did not receive Benlysta. "A clinical trial is ongoing to study Benlysta specifically in African Americans with lupus."[60] Development and approval of Benlysta "led the way for several promising new therapies now being tested in clinical trials."[61]

"Because of their disease severity and young age, lupus is a particular burden for children. Thus, any research that leads to improved understanding, treatment and quality of life in children has significant, lifelong implications."

–National Institutes of Health

"Other research is examining barriers that keep certain populations from complying with their prescribed medical treatment, which could contribute to worse disease outcomes, including disability and death in those populations."[62]

By most conservative estimates in 2007, there were 240,000 lupus patients living in the United States. During the same year, independent surveys suggested a prevalence as high as 1.5 million.[63] "Accurate estimates of the number of people who have a disease—as a whole and within specific groups—are important for a number of reasons, including understanding the disease and its impact; predicting groups and individuals who are most likely to develop lupus and, thus, are candidates for screening and preventive care; and providing care and services to people with the disease. Getting accurate estimates and updating them periodically can also enable researchers to determine if disease incidence is increasing and if so, start taking steps to understand why."[64]

"New concepts about the environment and rapid, sophisticated and high throughput technologies give hope to scientists and patients alike that many new discoveries will be made, and that these will be translated to transform the lives of lupus patients."[65]

Though lupus research has achieved advances in different areas such as genetics, disease process, and treatment, there are still many questions to be answered. "Doctors and scientists do not yet understand all of the factors that cause inflammation and tissue damage in lupus, and researchers are actively exploring them."[66] In *The Many Shades of Lupus*, NIH states that scientists are working on discovering more about causes and treatment of lupus. They are trying to solve several mysteries that surround the disease. Some of their questions are:[67]

- What causes lupus?
- Who is most susceptible to acquiring lupus and why?
- Why is lupus more prevalent among certain groups, such as African Americans, Asians, Hispanics/Latinos, and Native Americans?
- Why are cases in these groups often more severe?
- Why are women more likely than men to have the disease?
- What goes wrong in the immune system and why?

- How can we correct the way the immune system functions once something goes wrong?
- How do heredity and environment affect the disease process?
- What roles do factors like sunlight, stress, hormones, cigarette smoke, certain drugs, and infectious agents play in lupus?
- How can diagnostic procedures and treatment plans be improved?
- What treatment approaches will work best to lessen lupus symptoms?
- How can lupus be cured?

Some additional concerns I would like to see addressed are: more awareness initiatives, more accurate accounting for the number of lupus cases, more successful diagnostic procedures, prevention, better treatment plans with fewer and less potentially damaging side effects, more information on ways to predict and prevent flares, investigation of lupus as a possible underlying cause of other diseases, campaigns to attract more lupus healthcare specialists, and increased patient participation in research studies.

The hope is that a better understanding of roles that genetics, environment, and hormones play in the lupus diagnosis, as well as sufficient numbers of patients for clinical trials, will lead to earlier detection of lupus and better ways to treat and perhaps prevent the disease.[68] "There has never been more excitement in the government, academia and industry about lupus research and the prospects for improved diagnosis and therapies for this potentially devastating disease. Advances in technology as well as the development of partnerships—among the institutes, among centers and with patient advocacy groups and industry—promise to turn this excitement into new therapies to prevent the progression of lupus and its complications and perhaps even its onset."[69]

Records show that about ninety percent of people diagnosed with lupus are female. I am a female lupus patient, so opening doors for more research that would lead to a cure is extremely important to me. Additional efforts are needed to increase research because, as Dr. Wallace asserts, "Diseases of females are understudied by organized medicine." He goes on to say, "Research on lupus is also relatively underfunded compared to studies of other life-threatening diseases."[70]

"With research advances and better understanding of lupus, the prognosis for people with lupus today is far brighter than it was in the past. It is possible to have lupus and remain active and involved with life, family, and work. As current research efforts unfold, there is continued hope for new treatments, improvements in quality of life, and ultimately, a way to prevent or cure the disease. The research efforts of today may yield the answers of tomorrow, as scientists continue to unravel the mysteries of lupus."[71]

Participation of patients in clinical research is one of the best ways to advance new knowledge and contribute to the development of new treatments.[72] I agree wholeheartedly with this concept. My rheumatologist, Dr. Rosalind Ramsey-Goldman, conducts several lupus research studies at the Northwestern University in Chicago. I am participating in some of them. These are some of the studies in which I have participated: Fatigue and Lifestyle Physical Activities and SLE Study; SOLVABLE Heart and Bone Study; study examining the influence of lupus on the development of cardiovascular disease and osteoporosis; Systemic Lupus Erythematosus International Collaborating Clinics (SLICC)'s Registry for Atherosclerosis in SLE; and A Genetic Risk Profile in Longitudinal SLE Cohorts. I'm also involved in a study with the Arthritis Research Center Foundation National Data Bank for Rheumatic Disease.

What have *you* done lately to promote lupus awareness, to help fight for the cure? **MUCH MORE RESEARCH IS NEEDED. PLEASE GET INVOLVED!**

Appendix

Lupus Quiz

What do you now know about lupus?

The teacher in me does not allow you to leave this project without evaluating how much you've learned. Oh, that's right. For my results to be valid, I need to have given you a pretest also. Oh well, consider this a review.

Read each statement and decide if it is true or false.

1. Lupus causes the body's immune system to attack healthy cells.

2. Lupus is a very complex and unpredictable disease.

3. Scientists have discovered a cure for lupus.

4. It may take months or even years for doctors to diagnose lupus.

5. Lupus is **not** like cancer or HIV/AIDS.

6. Lupus can range from mild to life threatening.

7. Lupus may cause damage to virtually any tissue, organ, or system in the body.

8. Lupus is most common in women between the ages of 15 and 44.

9. Scientists report that possible causes of lupus may be linked to heredity, hormones, and environment.

10. Men, children, and older people cannot be diagnosed with lupus.

11. Lupus can be diagnosed with a simple blood test.

12. Lupus is contagious.

13. Lupus has many different symptoms, and each patient has a different set of symptoms.

14. It is estimated that there are at least 5 million people in the world and 1.5 million people in the U.S. who have some form of lupus.

Answers:

1.	true	6.	true	11.	false
2.	true	7.	true	12.	false
3.	false	8.	true	13.	true
4.	true	9.	true	14.	true
5.	true	10.	false		

Explanation of correct answers to the quiz may be verified by using the following sources:

- American Cancer Society
  *http://www.cancer.org/cancer/cancerbasics/
  what-is-cancer*
- American College of Rheumatology
  *http://www.rheumatology.org/Practice/Clinical/
  Patients/Diseases_And_Conditions/Systemic_
  Lupus_Erythematosus_(Lupus)*
- Lupus Foundation of America
  http://www.lupus.org/answers
- Lupus Research Institute
  *http://www.lupusresearchinstitute.org/lupus-
  facts/lupus-diagnosis*
- Lupus Society of Illinois
  http://www.lupusil.org/what-causes-lupus
- National Institute of Arthritis and Musculoskeletal and Skin Diseases
  *http://www.niams.nih.gov/health_info/lupus/
  lupus_ff.asp*
  *http://www.niams.nih.gov/about_us/Mission_
  and_Purpose/lupus_plan.asp#Pediatric_Lupus*
- U.S. Department of Health and Human Services
  *http://www.aids.gov/hiv-aids-basics/hiv-
  aids-101/what-is-hiv-aids*

Also used were NIH's *Handout on Health: Systemic Lupus
Erythematosus*, NIH's *The Many Shades of Lupus* pam-

phlet, the NIH Newsletter, *Coping With Lupus* by Robert H. Phillips, *The Lupus Book* by Daniel J. Wallace, and *Lupus: The Essential Clinician's Guide*, also by Wallace.

1. "In lupus, the body's immune system does not work as it should. A healthy immune system produces proteins called antibodies and specific cells called lymphocytes that help fight and destroy viruses, bacteria, and other foreign substances that invade the body. In lupus, the immune system produces antibodies against the body's healthy cells and tissues. These antibodies, called autoantibodies, contribute to the inflammation of various parts of the body and can cause damage to organs and tissues" (LSI website).

2. "Lupus is a very complex disease, and its cause is not fully understood" (NIH *Handout on Health*)." "Lupus is unpredictable because it is a disease of flares (symptoms worsen and you feel ill) and remissions (symptoms improve and you feel better)" (LFA website).

3. "Lupus is a chronic (lifelong) autoimmune disease" (LFA website). "At present, there is no cure for lupus" (NIH *Handout on Health*).

4. "Diagnosing lupus can be difficult. It may take months or even years for doctors to piece together the symptoms to diagnose this complex disease accurately" (NIH *Handout on Health*). Getting an accurate lupus diagnosis "...is often a very difficult and lengthy process, one that can take up to several years before the diagnosis is made" (*Coping With Lupus*, p 20).

5. "Lupus is not like or related to cancer or HIV/AIDS" (LFA website).

Lupus: Lupus is a chronic, autoimmune disease. Chronic means that the signs and symptoms tend to last longer than six weeks and often for many years. Autoimmune means that the body attacks itself. "A healthy immune system produces proteins . . . that help fight and destroy viruses, bacteria, and other foreign substances that invade the body."[2] If one has lupus, the immune system cannot tell the difference between foreign invaders and your body's healthy tissues. It then becomes overactive, creating autoantibodies that attack and destroy healthy tissue as well as the foreign invaders. These autoantibodies can cause inflammation, pain, and serious damage in various parts of the body. According to the NIH, any part of the body can be affected by lupus, including the kidneys, lungs, central nervous system, blood vessels, blood, and heart.[3] "Lupus is one of the cruelest, most mysterious diseases on earth. It strikes without warning, has unpredictable and sometimes fatal effects, lasts a lifetime, and has no known cure."[4] "Lupus is unpredictable because it is a disease of flares (symptoms worsen and you feel ill) and remissions (symptoms improve and you feel better)."[5]

Though the exact causes of lupus are unknown, many scientists believe that lupus develops as a response to a combination of internal and external factors including hormones, genetics, and the environment.[7] "Because symptoms vary from person to person, can come and go over time, and mimic other illnesses, lupus can be difficult to diagnose—and there is no definitive test for lupus."[14] Health effects of lupus might include, but are not limited to, heart attacks, strokes, seizures, kidney failure, and miscarriages.[6]

Cancer: Cancer is the general name for a group of more than 100 diseases. Although there are many kinds of cancer, all cancers start because abnormal cells grow out of control. Untreated cancers can cause serious illness and death. The body is made up of trillions of living cells. Normal body cells grow, divide to make new cells, and die in an orderly way. Cancer starts when cells in a part of the body start to grow out of control. Instead of dying, cancer cells continue to grow and form new, abnormal cells. Cancer cells can also invade (grow into) other tissues, something that normal cells can't do. Cells become cancer cells because of DNA (deoxyribonucleic acid) damage. DNA is in every cell and it directs all its actions. In a normal cell, when DNA is damaged the cell either repairs the damage or dies. In cancer cells, the damaged DNA is not repaired, but the cell doesn't die like it should. Instead, the cell goes on making new cells that the body doesn't need. These new cells all have the same damaged DNA as the first abnormal cell does. Sometimes the cause of the DNA damage may be something obvious like cigarette smoking or sun exposure. But it's rare to know exactly what caused any one person's cancer.

HIV/AIDS: "HIV" stands for Human Immunodeficiency Virus. An in-depth description of this term follows:

Human—This particular virus can only infect human beings.

Immunodeficiency—HIV weakens your immune system by destroying important cells that fight disease and infection. A "deficient" immune system can't protect you.

Virus—A virus can only reproduce itself by taking over a cell in the body of its host.

HIV is a lot like other viruses, including those that cause the "flu" or the common cold. But there is an important difference—over time, your immune system can clear most viruses out of your body. That isn't the case with HIV—the human immune system can't seem to get rid of it. That means that once you have HIV, you have it for life. We know that HIV can hide for long periods of time in the cells of your body and that it attacks a key part of your immune system—your T-cells or CD4 cells. Your body has to have these cells to fight infections and disease, but HIV invades them, uses them to make more copies of itself, and then destroys them. Over time, HIV can destroy so many of your CD4 cells that your body can't fight infections and diseases anymore. When that happens, HIV infection can lead to AIDS, the final stage of HIV infection. However, not everyone who has HIV progresses to AIDS. With proper treatment, called "antiretroviral therapy" (ART), you can keep the level of HIV virus in your body low.

6. Lupus can range from mild to life threatening, but symptoms can usually be managed with early, accurate diagnosis and proper treatment (NIH *Handout on Health*). Using research results from mortality studies that were reported by Abu-Shakra M. Urowitz in 1995, Wallace writes, "Currently, most patients with SLE

survive at least 20 years, although their quality of life is not always optimal" (*The Essential Clinician's Guide*, p. 93).

7. Lupus may affect many parts of the body, and everyone reacts differently (*The Many Shades of Lupus*). Lupus may cause damage to virtually any tissue, organ, or system in the body, especially the blood, blood vessels, brain or central nervous system, heart, joints, kidneys, lungs, and skin (NIH *Handout on Health*).

8. Anyone at any time can be diagnosed with lupus; however, nine out of ten cases are women. Ninety percent of lupus patients are women (LFA website). Lupus is most common in women between the ages of 15 and 44 (*The Many Shades of Lupus*). "Nearly 90% of persons with SLE are females…Most develop the disorder during their reproductive years" (*The Essential Clinician's Guide*, p. 12).

9. Scientists have not discovered what causes lupus. They report that some possibilities include the involvement of heredity, hormones, and environment. They also suggest evidence that sunlight, stress, and certain medicines may trigger symp-

toms in some people (*The Many Shades of Lupus*).

10. Men, children, and older people can also be diagnosed with lupus (*The Many Shades of Lupus*).

11. "No single test can identify lupus" (*The Many Shades of Lupus*). "Doctors use the American College of Rheumatology's 'Eleven Criteria of Lupus' to help make—or exclude—a diagnosis of lupus. Typically, four or more of the following criteria must be present to make a diagnosis of systemic lupus."

The Eleven Criteria:

Malar rash: butterfly-shaped rash across cheeks and nose

Discoid (skin) rash: raised red patches

Photosensitivity: skin rash as result of unusual reaction to sunlight

Mouth or nose ulcers: usually painless

Arthritis (nonerosive) in two or more joints, along with tenderness, swelling, or effusion. With nonerosive arthritis, the bones around joints don't get destroyed.

Cardio-pulmonary involvement: inflammation of the lining around the heart (pericarditis) and/or lungs (pleuritis)

Neurologic disorder: seizures and/or psychosis

Renal (kidney) disorder: excessive protein in the urine, or cellular casts in the urine

Hematologic (blood) disorder: hemolytic anemia, low white blood cell count, or low platelet count

Immunologic disorder: antibodies to double stranded DNA, antibodies to Sm, or antibodies to cardiolipin

Antinuclear antibodies (ANA): a positive test in the absence of drugs known to induce it.

12. "Lupus is not contagious, so you cannot catch lupus from someone or give lupus to someone" (LFA website). "…our research confirms that lupus cannot be spread from one person to another." (*The Lupus Book*, p. 48).

13. "Lupus has many different symptoms…" (LFA website). "Each person with lupus has slightly different symptoms that can range from mild to severe and may come and go over time" (NIH *Handout on Health*).

14. An estimated 1.5 million Americans and 5 million people worldwide have a form of lupus (LFA website). By most conservative estimates

in 2007, there were 240,000 lupus patients living in the United States. During the same year, independent surveys suggested a prevalence as high as 1.5 million. Further research is needed to ascertain the exact number of lupus cases.

References/Resources

Alliance for Lupus Research (ALR)

28 West 44th Street, Suite 501

New York, New York 10036

212-218-2840; 800-867-1743 (toll free)

info@lupusresearch.org

American Cancer Society

250 Williams Street NW

Atlanta, Georgia, 30303

800-227-2345

http://www.cancer.org/aboutus/howwehelpyou/
contactus/index

American College of Rheumatology (ACR)

2200 Lake Boulevard NE

Atlanta, Georgia 30319

Phone: (404) 633-3777; Fax: (404) 633-1870

acr@rheumatology.org

arhp@rheumatology.org

foundation@rheumatology.org

Centers for Disease Control and Prevention (CDC)

1600 Clifton Road

Atlanta, Georgia 30329-4027

800-CDC-INFO (800-232-4636)

http://wwwn.cdc.gov/dcs/RequestForm.aspx

Department Of Health and Human Services (DHHS)

HealthFinder is the DHHS site for consumer health information.

http://www.healthfinder.gov

Lupus Foundation of America, Inc. (LFA)

2000 L Street, N.W., Suite 410

Washington, DC 20036

202-349-1155; 800-558-0121

http://www.lupus.org

Lupus Research Institute (LRI)

330 Seventh Avenue, Suite 1701

New York, New York 10001

212-812-9881; 212-545-1843 (fax)

lupus@lupusny.org

http://www.lupusresearchinstitute.org

Lupus Society of Illinois (LSI)

525 W. Monroe St., Suite 900

Chicago, Illinois 60661-3793

312-542–0002; 800-258-7872 (toll free)

http://www.lupusil.org

MedlinePlus is the National Library of Medicine's Web site for consumer health information.

http://www.medlineplus.gov

National Institute of Arthritis and Musculoskeletal and Skin Diseases (NIAMS)

1 AMS Circle

Bethesda, Maryland 20892-3675

877-22-NIAMS (877-226-4267); TTY: 301-565-2966

NIAMSinfo@mail.nih.gov

http://www.niams.nih.gov

National Institutes of Health (NIH)

9000 Rockville Pike

Bethesda, Maryland 20892

301-496-4000; TTY 301-402-9612

NIHinfo@od.nih.gov

http://www.nih.gov

U.S. Food and Drug Administration (FDA)

10903 New Hampshire Avenue

Silver Spring, Maryland 20993

888-INFO-FDA (888-463-6332)

http://www.fda.gov

Books:

Daniel J. Wallace, MD. *The Lupus Book: A Guide for Patients and Their Families*, 5th Edition. New York, New York: Oxford University Press, 2013

Daniel J. Wallace, MD. *Lupus: The Essential Clinician's Guide.* New York, New York: Oxford University Press, 2008

Robert H. Phillips, PhD. *Coping With Lupus,* 4th Edition. New York, New York: the Penguin Group, 2012

Endnotes

1. National Institutes of Health, "Looking at Lupus: An Attack from Within," *NIH News in Health* (November 2011). http://newsinhealth.nih.gov/issue/Nov2011/Feature2

2. National Institute of Arthritis and Musculoskeletal and Skin Diseases. "Handout on Health: Systemic Lupus Erythematosus." http://www.niams.nih.gov/health_info/lupus

3. Ibid.

4. Lupus Society of Illinois. http://www.lupusil.org

5. Ibid.

6. Ibid.

7. National Institute of Arthritis and Musculoskeletal and Skin Diseases. *The Many Shades of Lupus: Information for Multicultural Communities.* NIH Publication No. 01–4958, August 2001.

8. Ginzler, Ellen, MD, and Jean Tayar, MD. "Systemic Lupus Erythematosus (Lupus)." American College of Rheumatology, February 2013. http://www.rheumatology.org/Practice/Clinical/Patients/Diseases_And_Conditions/Systemic_Lupus_Erythematosus_(Lupus)

9. National Institute of Arthritis and Musculoskeletal and Skin Diseases, "What is Lupus? Fast Facts," October 2009. http://www.niams.nih.gov/health_info/lupus/lupus_ff.asp

10. National Institute of Arthritis and Musculoskeletal and Skin Diseases. "Handout on Health: Systemic Lupus Erythematosus." http://www.niams.nih.gov/health_info/lupus

11. Ibid.

12. Ibid.

13. Lupus Society of Illinois, http://www.lupusil.org

14. Tucker, Lori, MD, and Sandra Watcher, RN, BSN. "Systemic Lupus Erythematosus in Children and Teens." American College of Rheumatology, July 2012.

https://www.rheumatology.org/Practice/Clinical/Patients/
Diseases_And_Conditions/Systemic_Lupus_
Erythematosus_in_Children_and_Teens

15. Ibid.

16. Ibid.

17. Lupus Foundation of America. "How Do I Explain Lupus to Others?" June 20, 2013. http://www.lupus.org/answers/entry/explaining-lupus

18. Lupus Foundation of America. "What Are the Common Symptoms of Lupus?" May 28, 2013. http://www.lupus.org/answers/entry/common-symptoms-of-lupus

19. Lupus Foundation of America. "Lupus Is a Cruel Mystery." http://www.cruelmystery.org

20. Lupus Society of Illinois, http://www.lupusil.org

21. National Institute of Arthritis and Musculoskeletal and Skin Diseases. "Handout on Health: Systemic Lupus Erythematosus." http://www.niams.nih.gov/health_info/lupus

22. Ginzler, Ellen, MD, and Jean Tayar, MD. "Systemic Lupus Erythematosus (Lupus)." American College of Rheumatology, February 2013. http://www.rheumatology.org/Practice/Clinical/Patients/Diseases_And_Conditions/Systemic_Lupus_Erythematosus_(Lupus)

23. National Institutes of Health, "Looking at Lupus: An Attack from Within," *NIH News in Health* (November 2011). http://newsinhealth.nih.gov/issue/Nov2011/Feature2

24. Lupus Foundation of America. "Statistics on Lupus." http://www.lupus.org/about/statistics-on-lupus

25. Lupus Foundation of America. "What Causes Lupus?" http://www.lupus.org/answers/entry/what-causes-lupus

26. Lupus Foundation of America. "How is Lupus Treated?" July 25,2013. http://www.lupus.org/answers/entry/how-is-lupus-treated

27. National Institute of Arthritis and Musculoskeletal and Skin Diseases. "Handout on Health: Systemic Lupus Erythematosus." http://www.niams.nih.gov/health_info/lupus

28. U.S. Food and Drug Administration. "FDA News Release: FDA Approves Benlysta to Treat Lupus." March 9, 2011. http://www.fda.gov/newsevents/newsroom/pressannouncements/ucm246489.htm

29. National Institute of Neurological Disorders and Stroke. "NINDS Neuromyelitis Optica Information Page." January 15, 2015. http://www.ninds.nih.gov/disorders/neuromyelitis_optica/neuromyelitis_optica.htm

30. National Institute of Arthritis and Musculoskeletal and Skin Diseases. "Handout on Health: Systemic Lupus Erythematosus." http://www.niams.nih.gov/health_info/lupus

31. National Institute of Arthritis and Musculoskeletal and Skin Diseases. *The Many Shades of Lupus: Information for Multicultural Communities*. NIH Publication No. 01–4958, August 2001.

32. Ibid.

33. National Institute of Arthritis and Musculoskeletal and Skin Diseases. "Handout on Health: Systemic Lupus Erythematosus." http://www.niams.nih.gov/health_info/lupus

34. Ginzler, Ellen, MD, and Jean Tayar, MD. "Systemic Lupus Erythematosus (Lupus)." American College of Rheumatology, February 2013. http://www.rheumatology.org/Practice/Clinical/Patients/Diseases_And_Conditions/Systemic_Lupus_Erythematosus_(Lupus)

35. National Institute of Arthritis and Musculoskeletal and Skin Diseases. "Handout on Health: Systemic Lupus Erythematosus." http://www.niams.nih.gov/health_info/lupus

36. MedlinePlus. "Colostomy." April 9, 2014. http://www.nlm.nih.gov/medlineplus/ency/article/002942.htm

37. MedlinePlus. "Mononucleosis." May 12, 2014. http://www.nlm.nih.gov/medlineplus/ency/article/000591.htm

38. Centers for Disease Control and Prevention. "About Epstein-Barr Virus (EBV)." January 6, 2014. http://www.cdc.gov/epstein-barr/about-ebv.html

39. MedlinePlus. "Sarcoidosis." May 30, 2013. http://www.nlm.nih.gov/medlineplus/ency/article/000076.htm

40. National Heart, Lung, and Blood Institute. "What Are the Signs and Symptoms of Sarcoidosis?" June 14, 2013. http://www.nhlbi.nih.gov/health/health-topics/topics/sarc/signs

41. MedlinePlus. "Sarcoidosis." May 30, 2013. http://www.nlm.nih.gov/medlineplus/ency/article/000076.htm

42. Lupus Research Institute. http://www.lupusresearchinstitute.org

43. American College of Rheumatology. "The Lupus Initiative." http://thelupusinitiative.org

44. Lupus Foundation of America. http://www.lupus.org

45. Lupus Society of Illinois. http://www.lupusil.org

46. National Institute of Arthritis and Musculoskeletal and Skin Diseases. *The Many Shades of Lupus: Information for Multicultural Communities.* NIH Publication No. 01–4958, August 2001.

47. Ginzler, Ellen, MD, and Jean Tayar, MD. "Systemic Lupus Erythematosus (Lupus)." American College of Rheumatology, February 2013. http://www.rheumatology.org/Practice/Clinical/Patients/Diseases_And_Conditions/Systemic_Lupus_Erythematosus_(Lupus)

48. Lupus Foundation of America. "Lupus Is a Cruel Mystery." http://www.cruelmystery.org

49. National Institute of Arthritis and Musculoskeletal and Skin Diseases. "The Future Directions of Lupus Research." August 2007. http://www.niams.nih.gov/about_us/Mission_and_Purpose/lupus_plan.asp

50. National Institute of Arthritis and Musculoskeletal and Skin Diseases. "Handout on Health: Systemic Lupus Erythematosus." http://www.niams.nih.gov/health_info/lupus

51. National Institute of Arthritis and Musculoskeletal and Skin Diseases. *The Many Shades of Lupus: Information for Multicultural Communities*. NIH Publication No. 01–4958, August 2001.

52. National Institute of Arthritis and Musculoskeletal and Skin Diseases. "The Future Directions of Lupus Research." August 2007. http://www.niams.nih.gov/about_us/Mission_and_Purpose/lupus_plan.asp

53. National Institute of Arthritis and Musculoskeletal and Skin Diseases. "Handout on Health: Systemic Lupus Erythematosus." http://www.niams.nih.gov/health_info/lupus

54. National Institute of Arthritis and Musculoskeletal and Skin Diseases. "The Future Directions of Lupus Research." August 2007. http://www.niams.nih.gov/about_us/Mission_and_Purpose/lupus_plan.asp

55. Ibid.

56. Ibid.

57. Ibid.

58. Ibid.

59. GlaxoSmithKline. "About BENLYSTA." http://www.benlysta.com/about/index.html

60. GlaxoSmithKline. "Risks and Side Effects." http://www.benlysta.com/risks-side-effects/index.html

61. National Institutes of Health, "Looking at Lupus: An Attack from Within," *NIH News in Health* (November 2011). http://newsinhealth.nih.gov/issue/Nov2011/Feature2

62. National Institute of Arthritis and Musculoskeletal and Skin Diseases. "Handout on Health: Systemic Lupus Erythematosus." http://www.niams.nih.gov/health_info/lupus

63. National Institute of Arthritis and Musculoskeletal and Skin Diseases. "The Future Directions of Lupus Research." August 2007. http://www.niams.nih.gov/about_us/Mission_and_Purpose/lupus_plan.asp

64. Ibid.

65. Ibid.

66. National Institute of Arthritis and Musculoskeletal and Skin Diseases. "Handout on Health: Systemic Lupus Erythematosus." http://www.niams.nih.gov/health_info/lupus

67. Ibid.

68. National Institute of Arthritis and Musculoskeletal and Skin Diseases. "The Future Directions of Lupus Research." August 2007. http://www.niams.nih.gov/about_us/Mission_and_Purpose/lupus_plan.asp

69. Ibid.

70. Wallace, Daniel J., MD. *The Lupus Book: A Guide for Patients and Their Families*, 5th Edition. New York, New York: Oxford University Press, 2013.

71. National Institute of Arthritis and Musculoskeletal and Skin Diseases. "Handout on Health: Systemic Lupus Erythematosus." http://www.niams.nih.gov/health_info/lupus

72. Ibid.